Don't Panic!

HOW TO USE YOGA TO SURVIVE THE COLLEGE EXPERIENCE

Bonnie Quiceno

ISBN-13: 9781539618522
ISBN-10: 1539618528
Library of Congress Control Number: 2016917515
CreateSpace Independent Publishing Platform
North Charleston, South Carolina

This book is for all of you struggling to keep your head above water as you climb the ladder toward being more educated and prepared to change the world in your chosen fields. It is my hope that through the suggestions made in this book you will understand how to use your body and your mind more effectively to excel in your work and still maintain a healthy, happy body. Here's to your success!

Acknowledgements

A special thank you to Farah Yamini and Sarah J. Hammill, without whom this book would never have become a reality. Thank you to my editor, Melanie Neale for her guidance through this process. To Krisi Keranova, thank you for your expertise with a camera, bringing out the best in me and for all of the photos to illustrate my words. Thank you Audre Carlin for always believing that I know what I'm talking about. Thank you Giselle for encouraging me to jump higher. Deep gratitude to Carla Hatchett Schwille for knowing how to solve every problem I ever had during this process and then proceeding to solve them. A huge thank you to my guru, Wynanda Jacoby, who has taught me more about yoga than I can express. Deepest gratitude to all of my FIU students/ family over the past 16 years. You shared everything about your lives, your struggles, your hopes and your fears with beautiful openness and honesty so that I might understand how better to guide you and ultimately share this information with others who stand to benefit from what you taught me. A big thank you also to all of the residents at Bay Oaks Assisted Living Facility. You taught me with your years and wisdom how to do yoga off the mat and in the most challenged of bodies. It is through this knowledge that I understand how to segue from the youth of the university students to the various stages of life and the importance of using yoga in every setting, not just on a mat in a yoga studio. Last, but not least, thank you to my mom who has always believed in me more than I believe in myself and saw the potential in me to write a book and for encouraging me to take action until I finally did, and to my husband who supports me even when he's not always sure what the method is behind the madness.

May you be enriched by this book as much as I have been enriched by you.
Om Shanti

Photography and Cover Photo by Krisi Keranova

Table of Contents

Disciamer

Before beginning any physical practice of yoga, you must consult with a medical professional regarding any health issues, injuries, or physical limitations. It is recommended that you read the entire book before practicing any of the techniques or physical postures. If you choose to practice any of the techniques or physical postures in this book you assume the risk of any resulting injury. This book is not intended to supplement or replace the guidance of a medical professional or that of a qualified teacher.

www.bonniequiceno.com
Facebook: Bonnie Quiceno
Instagram: @yogalove8
Twitter: @bonniequiceno
YouTube channel: Bonnie Quiceno

CHAPTER 1
What is Yoga?

"Yoga is the journey of the self, through the self, to the self."
~ THE BHAGAVAD GITA

Yoga is tying yourself into a knot and chanting a bunch of weird words. Ok, not really, but there is a popular misconception that yoga is that.

The root of the word yoga is "yug," meaning to join or bind, which doesn't give you much of an idea of what yoga is either. Some of the popular ideas are that yoga is exercise, yoga is meditating, yoga is stretching, and that yoga is relaxing. In an article by Shirley Archer, JD, MA in IDEA Health and Fitness Incorporated, it is said that "yoga is a physical activity that differs from physical exercise in that it offers mental, emotional and spiritual dimensions." So, which of these ideas is the correct one?

All of the above. There are physical postures that are considered to be exercise. You will stretch, you may meditate, and certainly yoga can be relaxing. There are a lot of ideas floating around about what yoga is, with good reason, because yoga is different things to different people.

Some of my students over the years have confessed that they were afraid to start a yoga practice because they thought it was a religion that may conflict with their own beliefs. Some people have thought yoga is a cult. When I first started teaching yoga, my mom came to visit. She enthusiastically went to every single class I taught every day. She was excited about her new discovery and related stories of yoga class to friends and family back home. Yoga was definitely not something practiced in my small Southern hometown and not readily understood by most people there. Finally, one day after a particularly exciting yoga story from my mom, the person on the other end said, "You're not getting into any witchcraft are you?" She was clearly uneducated on the topic.

The Paths of Yoga

To better understand what yoga is, let's take a look at the different paths of yoga.

1) **Raja Yoga: the royal path or yoga of meditation.**
   Through meditation, the mind is cleared and focus is sharpened in order to gain connection to the Divine.

2) **Karma Yoga: the yoga of action.**
   Your heart is purified because you are taught to act without thinking of receiving anything in return. Mother Teresa was a great example of a karma yogi.

3) **Jnana Yoga: the yoga of knowledge or wisdom.**
   Jnana means knowledge, and this type of yoga refers to union due to pure knowledge. An aspirant would study sacred texts to gain the knowledge to release one from bondage. Through deep study of sacred texts, you no longer perceive a separation between the Self and the Divine.

4) **Bhakti Yoga: devotional.**
   Practitioners are motivated by the power of love.
   Chanting and singing are a big part of this path of yoga.

5) **Hatha Yoga: the yoga of physical postures, called asanas, or exercises as we tend to view them in the West.**
   In some texts about yoga, hatha yoga is not included as one of the paths of yoga. But in others, it is. Hatha yoga is what we Westerners most frequently think of when we hear the word yoga.

Why Hatha Yoga Is Useful For College Students

Thousands of years ago when people tried to sit and meditate they were just like us. Their minds wandered. Their backs hurt. They fell asleep. They had gas, and all of the same things we experience. To combat these challenges, they decided they needed to develop a way to solve the issues in the body that were distracting the mind from the desired result of peaceful meditation. And so hatha yoga was born.

There are many forms of hatha yoga. There is Ashtanga Vinyasa, Sivananda, Iyengar, Bikram, Anusara, and the list goes on. But they all fall under the general heading of hatha yoga. There are many facets to yoga. You may choose a spiritual path, but you may also choose a path of physical wellbeing.

Hatha yoga is designed to tone every part of your body from the inside out so you can sit and meditate as long as you want without feeling discomfort in your body. What if you could do this so you could study without being uncomfortable? Imagine how much more focused you could be. And how much better use you could make of your study time. Let's think about why we should and how we can make that happen.

CHAPTER 2
The Delightful Effects of Not Moving Enough

"Yoga is 99% practice and 1% theory."
~ SRI K. PATTABHI JOIS

College Degrees and Healthy Lifestyles

et's be honest. Earning a college degree is probably not the easiest thing you will ever do in your life. You have classes, lab, homework, research, group projects, and that's just school. On top of that, many of you are working full, or at least part-time jobs, and then have families that also deserve your time and attention. So where are you in all of this mash up of things to do? You might find yourself and your personal needs coming in last, or, worse yet, not at all.

Unfortunately, during their time as undergraduates, too many college students develop health issues or lifestyle patterns that over time cause them to develop health issues.

Challenges a College Student Faces
Challenge 1: A Sedentary Lifestyle

There may be a number of challenges that you face while you are trying to attain a higher education. There are two major challenges that are a common denominator for everyone whether they are a science, engineering, or arts and humanities major. The first is likely to be a sedentary lifestyle, i.e. not moving around enough.

Most college studies involve sitting in lecture classes, sitting to do research, sitting to study and sitting to drive or ride to school and work. After a while your body begins to develop a feeling of always being in the shape of a chair. There are many studies showing the unpleasant side effects of not using your body enough. They include things like:

- Pain
- Difficulty concentrating
- Poor sleep
- Inability to perform your best
- Grades dropping
- Anxiety/panic attacks
- Weight gain
- Poor health

To understand the less-than-desirable effects of not moving around enough, let's look at the iliopsoas muscle. The iliopsoas muscle is located mostly deep in your abdomen and is the boss in charge of all forward bending. When we are sitting, we are essentially bending forward. The iliopsoas becomes hypertonic or chronically shortened. Over time, it has a hard time lengthening out again.

Because of the location of the iliopsoas, deep in your abdomen, too much tightness may also cause tension or squeezing on other parts of your abdomen, including your intestines and other abdominal organs. This translates to you as low back pain, hip pain, poor digestion, and sluggishness in other organs as well. On top of that, humans are creatures of habit—the less we move, the less we want to move. Do you see where I'm heading?

The problem with sitting is that muscles were made to be used. They have a use-it-or-lose-it mentality. They crave movement and when they don't get it they begin to whimper. At first it's softly. The first consequence is soft-tissue stagnancy. The worst manifestation is decubitus ulcers, more commonly known as bedsores. Certainly you aren't likely to get a bedsore from sitting at your desk studying for hours, but in order to survive and thrive your muscles will begin to scream for both physical and neurological stimulation. You get up and go to the bathroom or to class which is just enough to stop the tissues from becoming completely necrotic (which, ironically, sounds a lot like neurotic), but they get sickly anyway. Especially the shoulders, the back and the hips, which stiffen to the point that the pelvis loses mobility and circulation.

Maybe it's time to ask yourself if your chair could be slowly killing you. I know it sounds drastic, but there is a rather mountainous pile of research showing up everywhere indicating that this might just be the case. There are articles appearing everywhere from the Wall Street Journal ("Sitting For More Than 3 Hours A Day Cuts Life Expectancy") to the NY Times ("Is Sitting A Lethal Activity?") to Popular Science with "7 Ways Sitting Will Kill You." On top of it all, the more you sit, the more you feel like you want to sit.

The more you keep sitting, the more aches and pains you develop in your body and the harder it becomes to move. The will to move keeps decreasing and then you graduate and land a job out in the big, bad "real world" and you have already developed an unhealthy pattern of sitting too much and not taking care of yourself. Suddenly you realize graduating did nothing to help you have more time for taking care of yourself and voila! You are on a fast track to losing your physical and mental health. Is this what you signed up for when you chose to go to school? If it is, by all means carry on with your plans. If it's not what you wanted for yourself, then what on earth do you plan on doing about it?

Challenge 2: Not Enough Time

The second big challenge in school is a lack of time. School alone requires a lot of time devoted to completing all of the coursework. Add to that needing to work to pay for school, housing, food, etc., and there is precious little time to take care of yourself.

Exercise and eating well are usually the first to go. I often get to know students at the university where I teach, even if they don't come to my yoga classes. Many of them end up telling me their stories.

Rodrigo (name changed) was one such student. He came in as an eager freshman ready to conquer the world. He wasn't particularly athletic, but he was young and in okay shape physically. Within a few weeks of fall semester's busy schedule, he was beginning to lose steam.

I talked to him about how yoga could help him balance his hectic life, but he just couldn't grasp how one more thing on his plate was going to help him. We bumped into each other from time to time throughout the years and he remained overwhelmed, barely keeping his head above water, but he maintained really good grades. I watched as he gained weight, got some premature gray hairs, and looked more and more stressed. In his fourth year of school, he told me he had been to see his doctor and had been told he was borderline diabetic.

He never took my advice during school about trying yoga, or something physical to help him through his difficult journey. He graduated with a good GPA and a body that was a ticking time bomb, waiting to explode into full-blown chronic health issues.

He contacted me about three years after he graduated and wanted to know if I could give him guidance on finding a good yoga teacher in his city. He had landed his dream job but was miserable because of his weight and other health issues. After joining the workforce for a few years, he realized that work was going to last for a really long time and he could no longer maintain the stamina for it if he continued to ignore the needs of his body.

Yoga During College Life = Healthy Habits for Life

A study looking at 2012 college students showed that 79 percent of college students were aged 18-24. The average life expectancy of American adults in 2012 was 78.8 years old. That's fifty odd years of life after undergraduate studies that you have left to live.

How you do want to feel in those next fifty or so years? Do you want to wait until retirement to get your life together in such a way that you feel great and do everything you want to do?

Certainly, spending time on your studies is super important and so is making excellent grades. So is your mental, physical and emotional health. What if you could have it all? That's what I'm proposing you learn to do with this book. Learn ways to keep your body, mind and spirit healthy while studying.

In the following chapters you will learn the 3 yoga keys to staying healthy while moving through school and all of its challenges with a lot more ease. Your college years will be healthier and happier and so will the entire rest of your life because you will develop habits that lead to a healthier life.

But before we move on to those three keys, I invite you to use the next pages to map out your intentions and priorities to create the best 50 or so years you possibly can. It is important to know where you are going, but it is crucial to have directions of how to get there. Imagine if you decided you wanted to take a trip to the beach but you had never been before. You may or may not make it to the beach if you had no idea what roads to take to get there. Most of you would never try to get to the beach without directions, yet that is exactly what many people do with their lives. Deciding you want to be an engineer is not enough. You must first determine what steps you need to take to get the college degree that states that you are qualified. Then you must take steps to get a job, keep it and still live a happy, healthy life. The next pages are for you to create your road map for your life.

Begin by listing your intentions for school, work, you and family (or any priorities you choose) in 3 categories: short term, medium term, and long term. Next, decide how long is the timespan for each category. For school, you may want to do two separate lists, one for individual semesters and another for the rest of your college career.

Finally, fill out the pages to the best of your ability. You may not know every detail right away. This should be a work in progress that you return to again and again to continually evolve. Therefore, it won't matter if some things are really clear and others are a bit muddy in your mind and on the paper. Just fill out everything to the best of your ability and with the passage of time you will change and rearrange things to suit you as you see more clearly what you need to do.

Intentions and Priorities

Intentions and Priorities

Intentions and Priorities

Intentions and Priorities

Intentions and Priorities

Intentions and Priorities

Intentions and Priorities

Intentions and Priorities

Intentions and Priorities

Intentions and Priorities

Intentions and Priorities

Intentions and Priorities

CHAPTER 3

Body, Mind, Breath Connection: Powerful Tools for Academic Success

"Yoga allows you to rediscover a sense of wholeness
in your life, where you do not feel like you are
constantly trying to fit broken pieces together"
~ B.K.S. IYENGAR

There are three basic components that are essential ingredients to a successful hatha yoga practice. But first, what do I mean by successful? Does success in your practice mean you can perform every posture or asana with ease? No! Success means you achieved the desired result. Let's set our intention as this: learn to use yoga to get through school with ease, resulting in a successful graduation. With that intention in mind, let's look at the three basic components needed. They are:

- Body
- Breath
- Mind

Do you have all of those already? I'm pretty sure you do! Now the trick is to learn how to use them effectively. Let's think about each of them and how they might be connected to each other. Once you have learned them in this order, feel free to use them in any order that serves your needs at the moment. We normally consider our bodies first, our minds second, and our breath last (if at all). One of my goals with this book is to get you to think of these three things with equal importance and give them equal attention in your yoga practice and in your life.

1. **Body:**

   You use your body to get from place to place and do the physical things you want to do, whether it's walking, jumping, swimming, hugging, studying, driving or anything else. Your mind and your breath help your body do these movements. But have you ever thought about how to use your body more effectively for your studies?

2. **Breath:**

   Breathing is the first thing you do when you come into the world and the last thing you do on your way out. What about all of the breaths between the first one and the last one?

   Maybe it's a good idea to pay attention to them and what breath does besides keep us alive. The next time you're stressed or angry, notice your breath. Most likely you're holding your breath a lot, and when you do breathe, it's very shallow and quick through your mouth. The next time this happens, try breathing slowly and deeply, through your nose only.

3. **Mind:**

   Of course you have a brain to think, reason, make decisions, and so on. But remember, there are also subconscious thoughts: the voice inside your head and the so-very-subtle thoughts and belief systems that run the show in such a way that you don't even know they are there. You may find yourself doing something without realizing what you were doing, and without a conscious decision to do so. Did you know that you can control your thoughts to help you study? Even the most subtle thoughts? Notice your body and your mind getting more relaxed. Did you know that you can use your breath to control your mind and your body? Did you know your breath is the master key to everything you do and that just by learning simple breathing techniques you could improve your study time and your performance on exams?

It is impossible to affect one of these three without affecting the others. The ancient yogis knew this and learned how to use it to their benefit. I call this the Body, Mind, Breath Connection. And if you learn to use it effectively, you will find all of your university challenges much less difficult. Then you can carry it into your life beyond school and continue to be successful in all of your endeavors. This is a valuable tool you need to get you through school and beyond.

CHAPTER 4
The Body

"Do your practice and all is coming."
~ SRI.K. PATTABHI JOIS

Yoga Asanas While Studying

"But I don't have time to go to yoga classes!" If I had a dollar for every time someone told me this in my seventeen years of teaching at a university, I would have a small fortune by now. And you know what? I get it. I really do. I was a college student too and finding time to eat was a challenge on many days. Luckily for me, I was a theater major with a dance emphasis, so I was required to move for much of my coursework. It was this movement that got me through a lot of the stress and tension. I knew nothing about yoga at that time, but boy if I had! Knowing what I know now about also using the breath and the mind would have been invaluable. I'm pretty sure having those tools to add to the physical body training in my college days would have made me invincible!

But if you don't have time to come to yoga classes or they aren't available to you, how can you work yoga exercises into your daily routine? At the university where I teach, we have "Yoga Study Hall" each semester in the week before finals. Here, I teach students how doing movement while studying can clear brain fog, prevent physical discomfort and integrate your studies into your memory in a way that sedentary study time doesn't.

Using Yoga Study Hall as a Model

Students bring books, laptops, or whatever they need to help them study. We begin the class seated on our mats, with study tools beside us. Each person briefly states their intention of what they want to accomplish during our hour and a half together. We then begin with about ten minutes of yoga practice, breathing, getting centered, grounding, and relaxing the nervous system. And then, its stop, drop and study. I give ten or fifteen minutes of study time and then we take a yoga break. We continue this way until we finish an hour and a half. I usually mix up the length of yoga time and study time to accommodate everyone's needs, which brings me to an important point.

How long can you study before you lose focus? If you aren't sure, pay attention, because most everyone has a time span that they can maintain focus. Notice things like a wandering mind, not retaining study material, getting on social media instead of studying, and all of the other behaviors that warn you that you are losing focus. Remember that the amount of time can vary depending on what you're studying. Using me as a model, if I'm studying something like what herbs are good to cure the common cold, I'm good for half an hour. If I'm studying something mathematical in nature, I'm only good for about five minutes!

Set an alarm just before your burnout time. For example, if you max out at fifteen minutes, set your alarm at thirteen or fourteen minutes, so that you have time to wrap it up before your study brain expires.

If you keep pushing past your attention span, it's usually counterproductive. It's better to take a break and come back to it. You'll accomplish more in the long run. This is where your yoga practice comes in. Study for as long as you can concentrate fully and then stop and do some yoga. Let me show you some simple ways to incorporate yoga into your study time.

At the end of this chapter there are blank pages. I recommend you use them to note how you feel before doing the exercises and how you feel after doing them. One way is to note on a scale of 1 to 10, with 1 representing feeling your worst and 10 representing feeling your best. Jotting down which postures you did may also be useful.

It is human nature to forget how we felt 5 minutes ago, an hour ago, or yesterday, let alone a month ago or last semester. Writing down how you feel before and after will help you see the benefits of the suggestions in this book as you use it. It will also be invaluable in years to come, if you've fallen out of the habit of using these tools, to remind yourself of the benefits you experienced. That can be a powerful tool to help your future self move back into regular usage of this book.

Using Your Desk and Wall as a Yoga Tool:

1) **Desk Down Dog**
   - Standing with feet hips-width apart, place your hands on top of your desk.
   - Walk your feet back until your spine is parallel to the floor or as close as is possible for you.
   - Take three to five deep breaths.
   - Walk your feet slowly back in, on an inhale, until you're standing straight.

Desk Down Dog

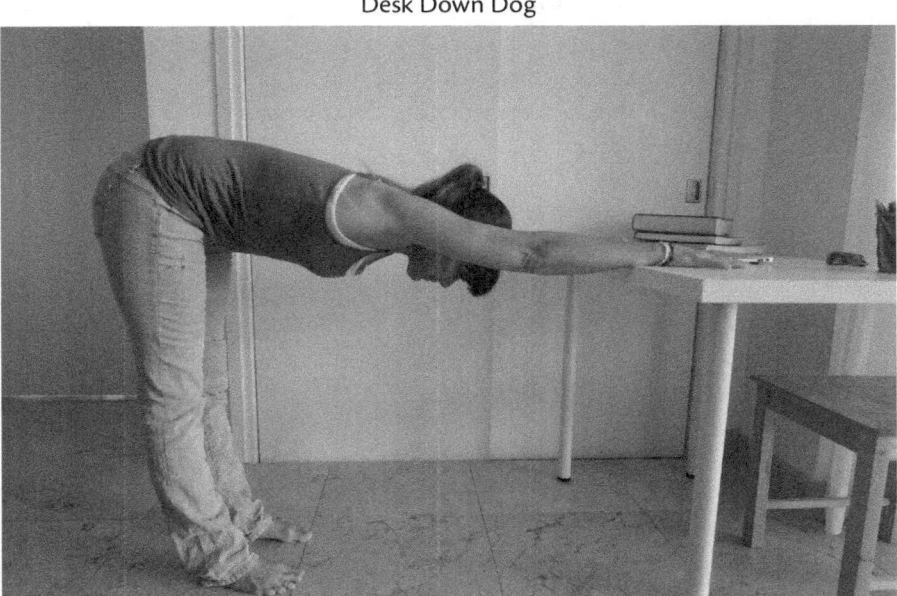

Hands on desk. Spine parallel to floor.

Benefits: *This will release tension in your lower back as well as between the shoulder blades and in your neck. It will also stretch the back of your legs, which tighten up from sitting and eventually can cause low back pain and a forward bent posture. As a result, you will get more blood flow to your brain from releasing the neck and shoulders and to your legs from releasing tight hamstrings. Blood to your brain means better use of study time, which means you learn more and get better grades. More blood flow to your legs means less physical discomfort, resulting in fewer distractions from body aches, which translates into better focus while studying.*

2) **Standing Half-Frog**
   - Stand with your left side toward your desk.
   - Hold onto your desk with your left hand.
   - Bend your right knee.
   - Clasp your right foot or your ankle with your right hand and pull it in toward the back of your hip.
   - You should feel a stretch in the front of your right thigh, in the quadriceps area.
   - Release your foot gently back to the floor.
   - Turn around to face the opposite direction and repeat the same thing with your left foot.

Standing Half-Frog

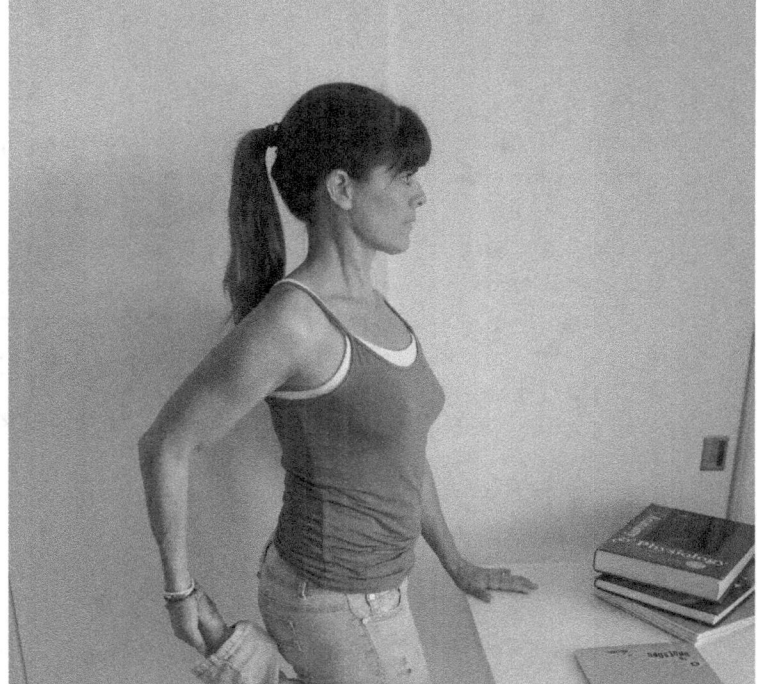

One hand on desk. Pull opposite foot to buttock.

Benefits: *The quadriceps are stretched and the hip flexors are released. Again, we have more blood flow to the areas addressed, resulting in less physical discomfort, better focus when studying and a healthier, happier body.*

3) **Tree Pose**
   - Stand with your back lightly touching a wall. Even if you have a yoga practice and do tree pose without the wall, try using it. Actually touching the wall will remind you to keep your spine straight and tall and help shift you out of your head and back into your body. Studying brings you very much into a head space, which is necessary, but needs to be balanced by coming back into the body so you don't lose touch with the needs of your physical body.
   - Bring your feet hips-width apart and turn them facing straight forward.
   - Fix your gaze on a spot that won't move and keep it there.
   - Pick up your right foot and place it against the inside of the left thigh, calf, or ankle. (Never rest your foot on your knee.)
   - The heel of the lifted foot is turned upward and the toes are turned downward, towards the floor.
   - Place your hands together at the center of your chest, and press your palms together.
   - This hand position helps you find your center and hold your balance.
   - Take three to five slow, deep breaths.
   - Release your right foot and repeat with the left foot.

Tree Pose

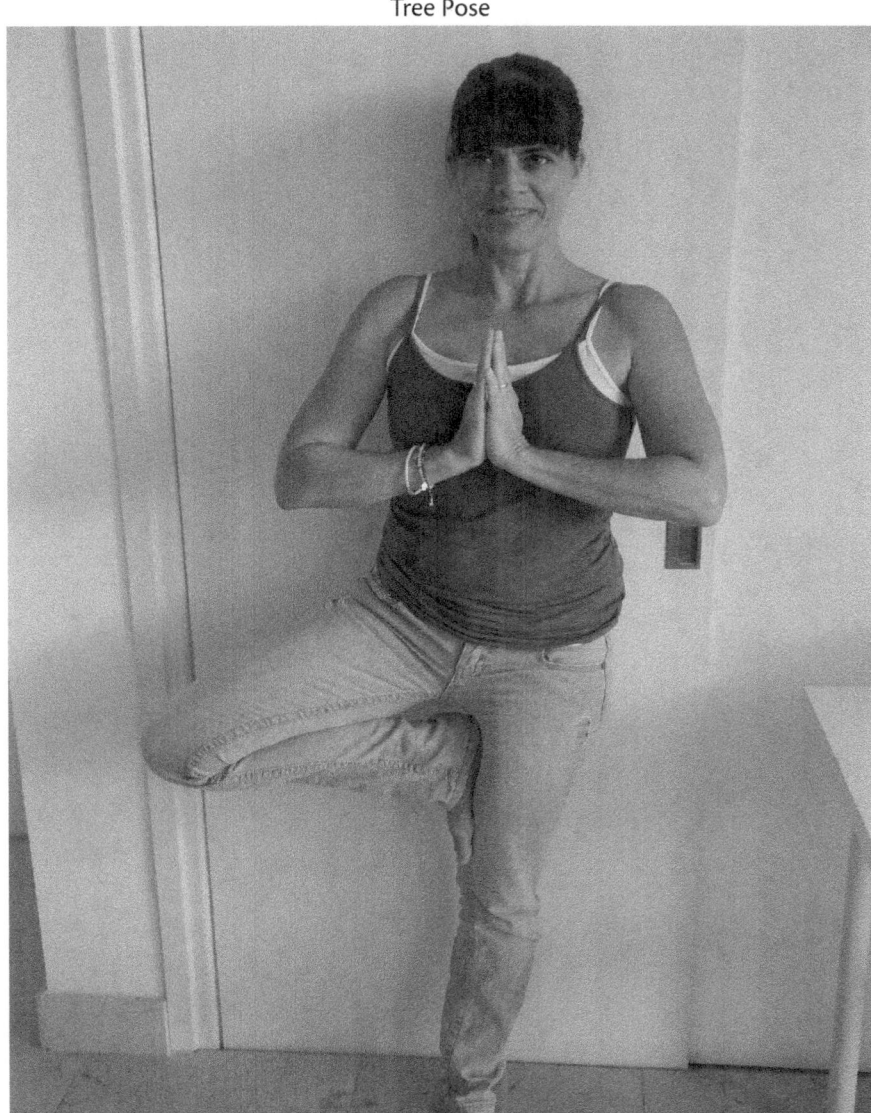

One foot on inside, opposite leg.

Tree Pose

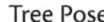

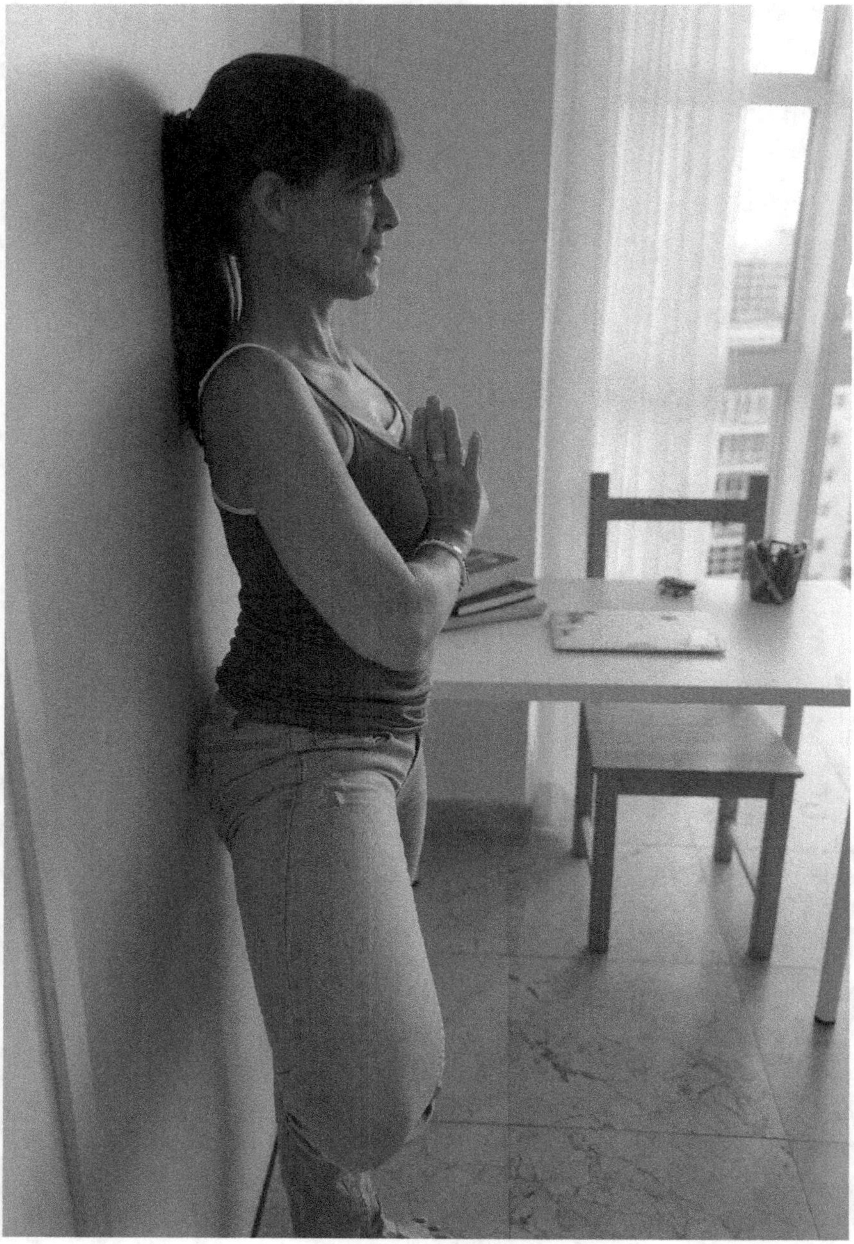

Back against wall.

Benefits: *Tree pose develops focus and the ability to see challenging situations through to the end, and allows the spine to realign. A properly aligned spine creates a healthy nervous system, which brings health to the entire body. Better focus means better grades, which translates to scholarships, awards, and offers for your dream job after school is done.*

4) **Forward Bend with an Amped-up Enhanced Hamstring Stretch**
   - With your back resting firmly against a wall, walk your feet forward a foot or so away from the wall.
   - Keep the back of your body resting against the wall.
   - Inhale deeply through your nose and lengthen your spine.
   - As you exhale, allow your body to fall forward over your legs, keeping your spine as long and straight as possible.
   - Let your arms drop toward the floor, or place them on your thighs or shins if you need to make the stretch less intense.
   - Hang there for three to five deep breaths then slowly roll up your spine.

Forward Bend with an Amped-Up Hamstring Stretch

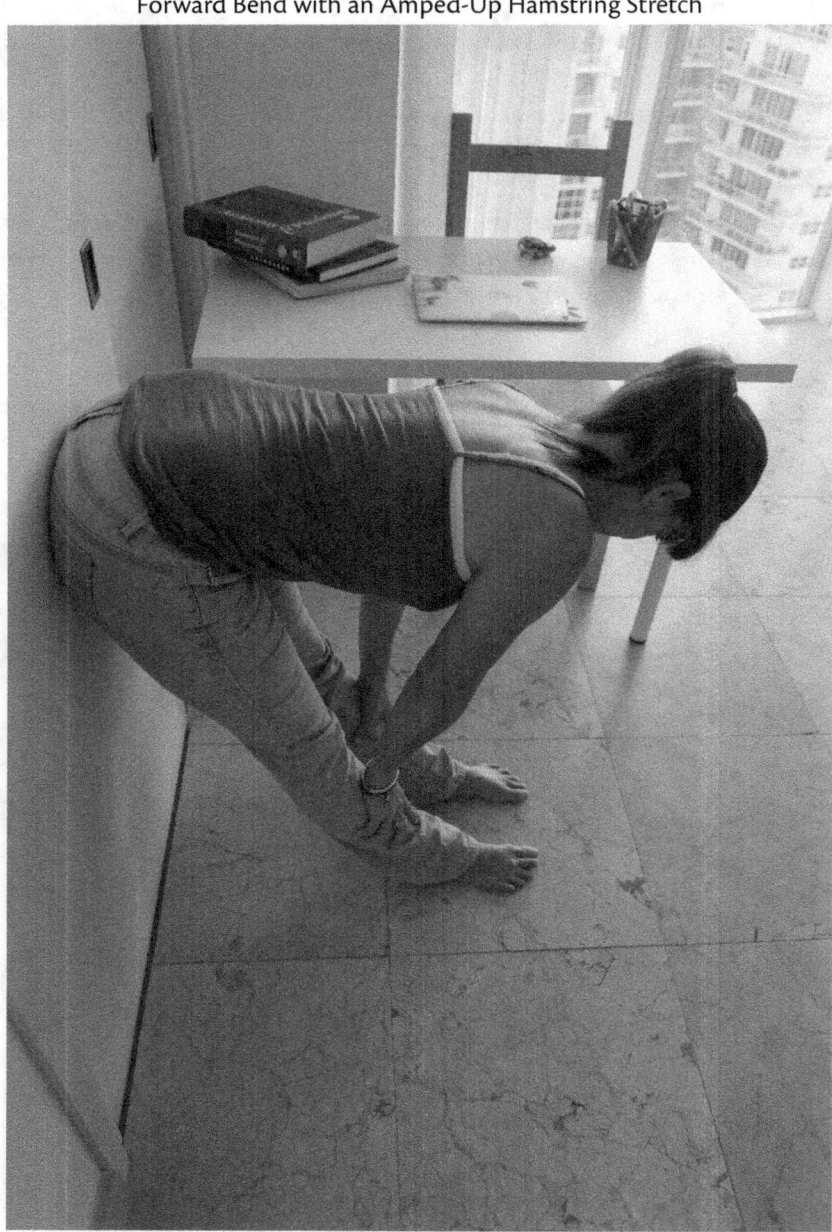

Feet away from wall, buttocks against wall.

Forward Bend with an Amped-Up Hamstring Stretch

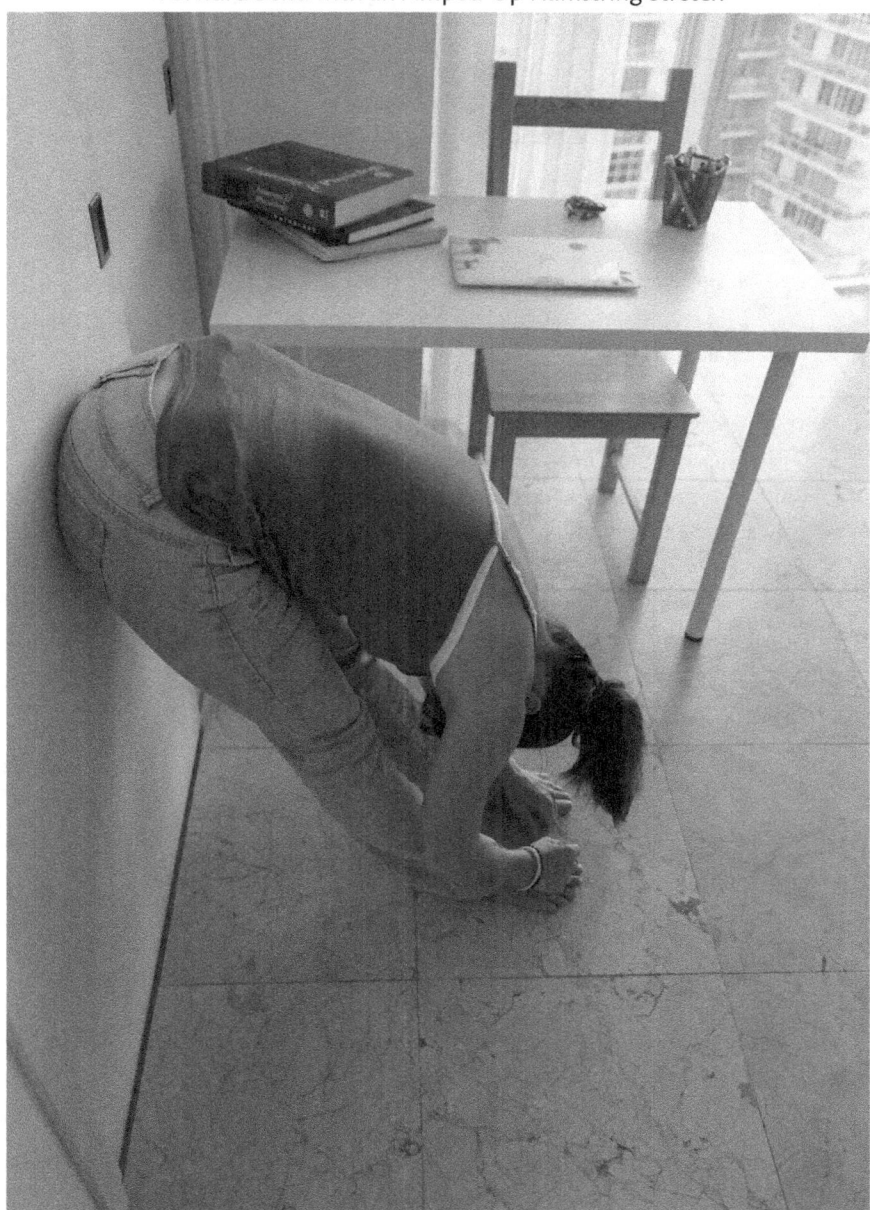

Bend forward.

Benefits: _This exercise will calm your nervous system and get more blood to your_
brain.

It's very useful when you're stressed, or when you've been studying for a while, and you
have that brain fog feeling that makes it difficult to think. It stretches your hamstrings, giving
your legs more mobility, and releases low back tension. This means you will study more effec-
tively, which results in better grades, plus you'll have a healthier back.

5) **Shoulder Opener**
   - Stand with your left side against the wall, feet hips-width apart.
   - Bring your left hand back behind you, with the inside of your palm against the wall.
   - Slide your hand up as high as possible against the wall behind you.
   - Keep your hips and shoulders perpendicular to the wall.
   - Breathe super deep breaths for three to five rounds.
- Allow the tension and strain to leave from your chest and shoulders as you reverse the hunched over position that comes from poring over books and sitting at a computer.
- Slowly slide the hand back down the wall until it's relaxed at your side again.
- Turn around and repeat with the right arm.

Shoulder Opener

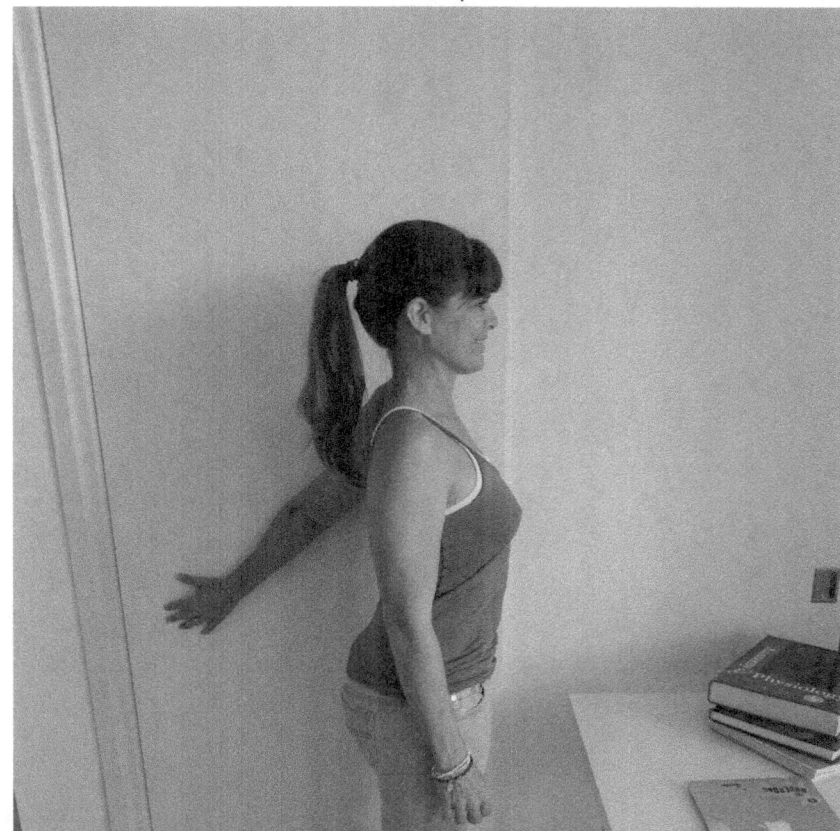

Stand with side to wall.

Shoulder Opener

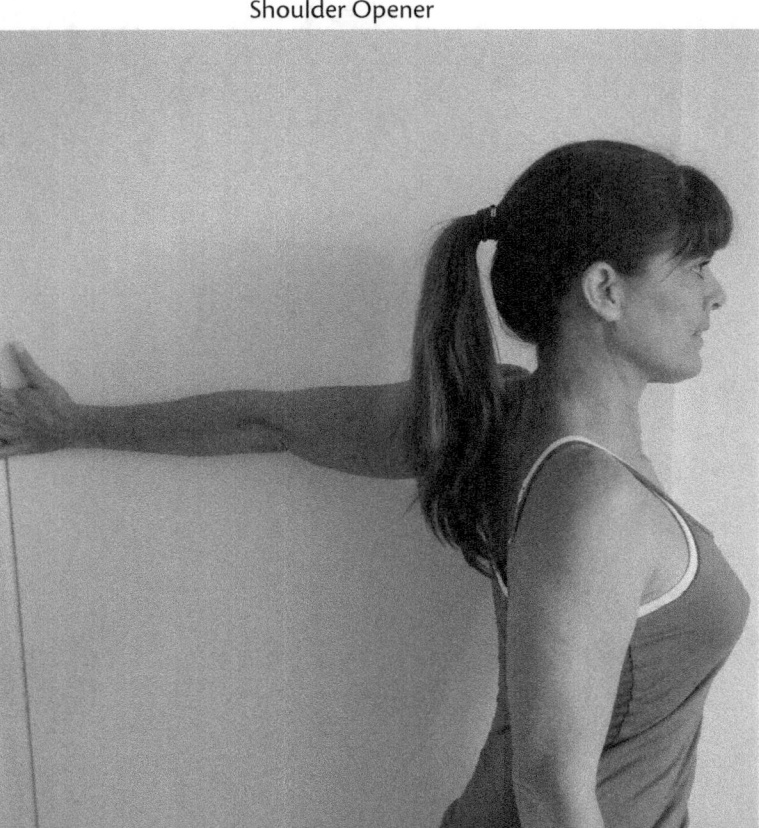

Reach back and up. Palm against wall.

Benefits: *This releases tension in the shoulders and upper half of your back. It also helps reverse the hunched-over-a -computer-look and helps bring circulation into the shoulders arms, hands, and fingers. It opens the heart and lungs, helping to keep them healthy, and oxygenates your entire body. This creates both short- and long-term health.*

Using Your Chair as a Yoga Tool:

1) **Seated Tadasana, or Chair Mountain Pose**
   - Sit near the edge of your chair, with your feet planted hips-width apart, flat on the floor.
   - Even out your weight on both sitting bones, with equal weight on both sides.
   - Lengthen your spine by sitting straight and tall.
   - Let your shoulders relax down and away from your ears.
   - Actively press your feet into the floor, then reach up, through the top of your head.
   - You should feel as if your spine is getting longer and more spacious.
   - Take three to five deep breaths in and out through your nose.

Seated Tadasana, or Chair Mountain Pose

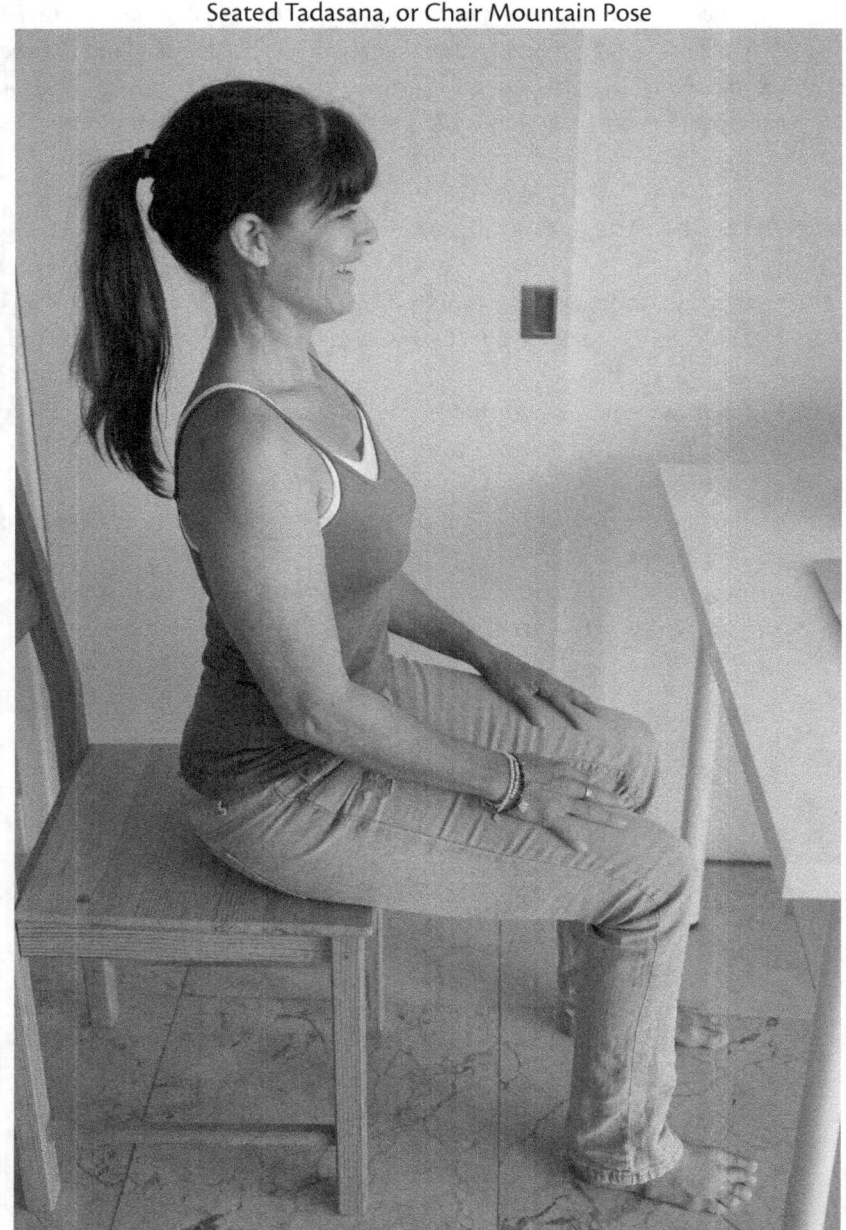

Sit on edge of chair. Press feet into floor, spine long.

Benefits: _This posture reverses a sagging spine from too much sitting, rejuvenates the upper body, and allows more blood flow to the brain. It activates the legs and helps you maintain better posture with your legs even when seated, and teaches you to align your posture. An aligned posture leads to a healthier nervous system, a more nourished brain, and the ability to use your brain more fully and effectively._

2) **Neck Saver**
   - Stay in the seated Tadasana you just created.
   - Inhale look up, exhale look down
   - Inhale your head to center, exhale look right.
   - Inhale head to center, exhale look left.
   - Inhale look up right, exhale look down left. Your head is now moving diagonally.
   - Inhale, look up left, exhale look down right.
   - Inhale bring your face to center. Imagine your nose is in the center of a huge clock.
   - Breathe deeply in and out through your nose as you look up to 12 o'clock, 1 o'clock, 2 o'clock, and so on until you work your way back up to 12 o'clock.
   - Reverse and go around counterclockwise, breathing deeply.

Neck Saver

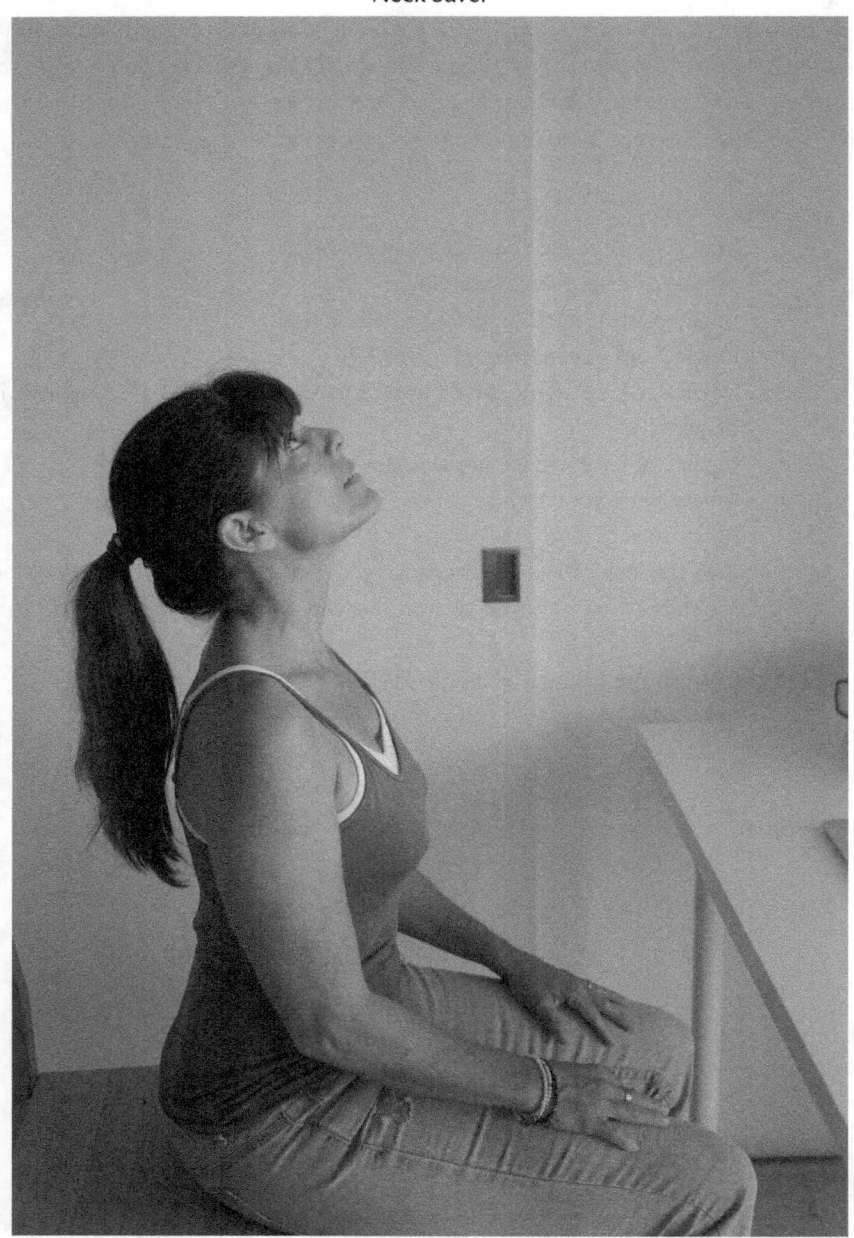

Inhale. Lift face up. ↑

Neck Saver

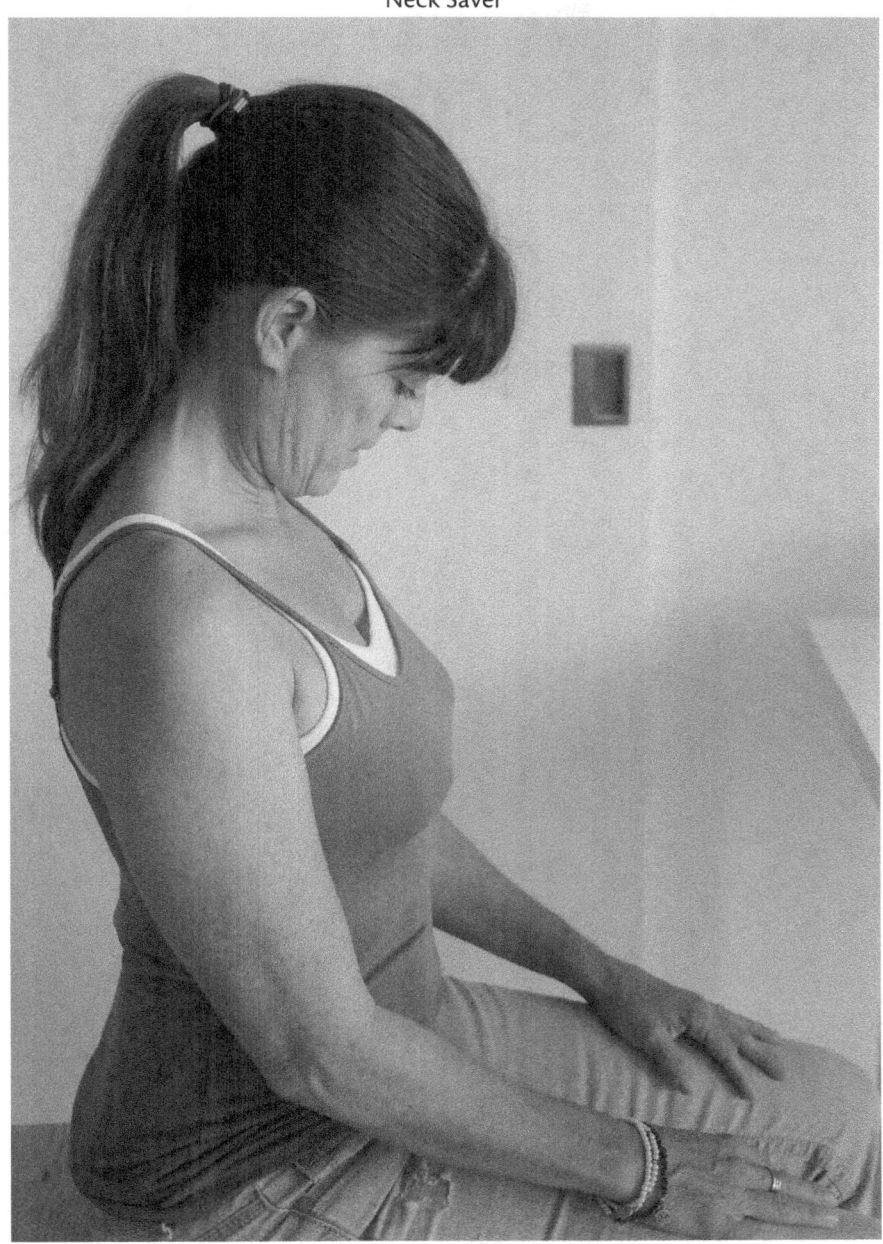

Exhale. Drop face down. ↓

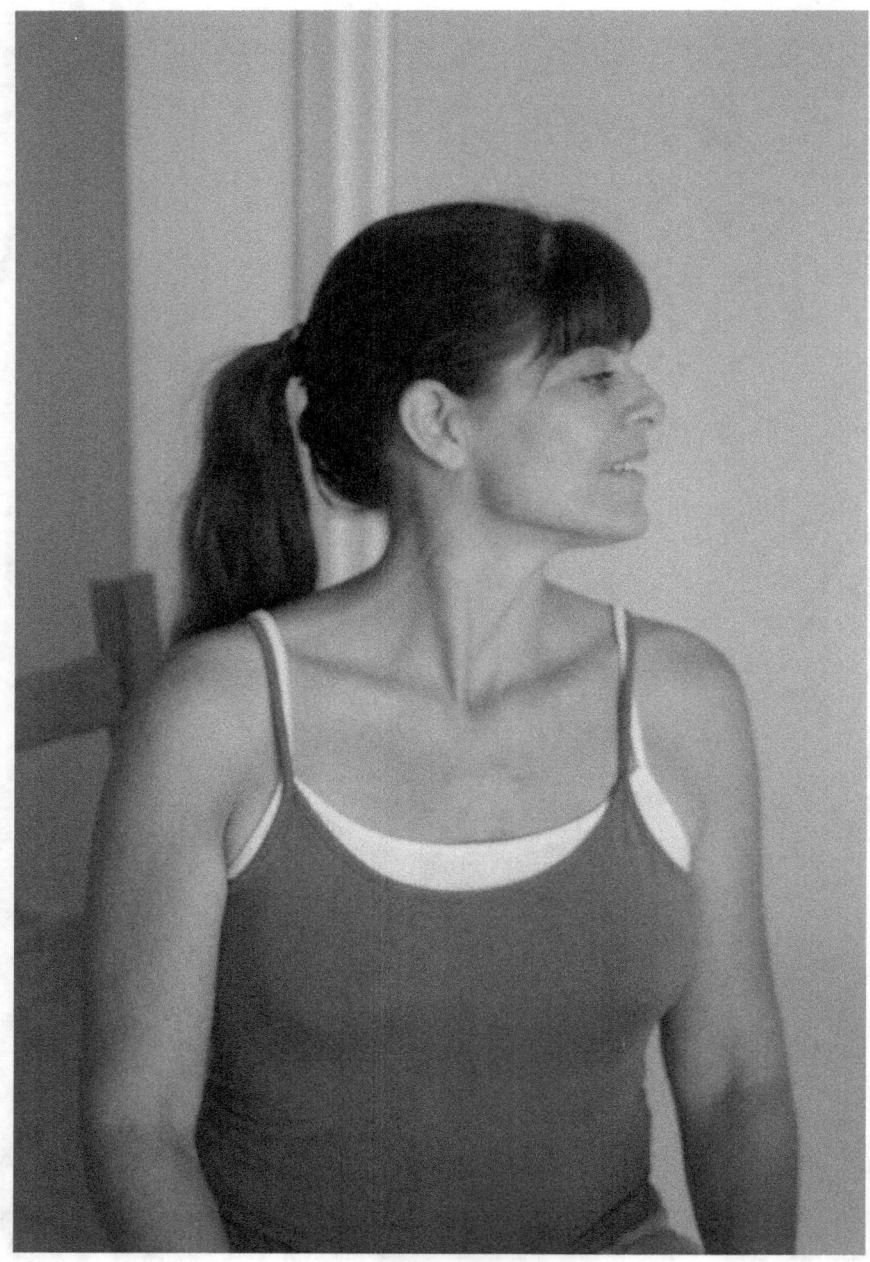

Inhale. Turn face right. ➜

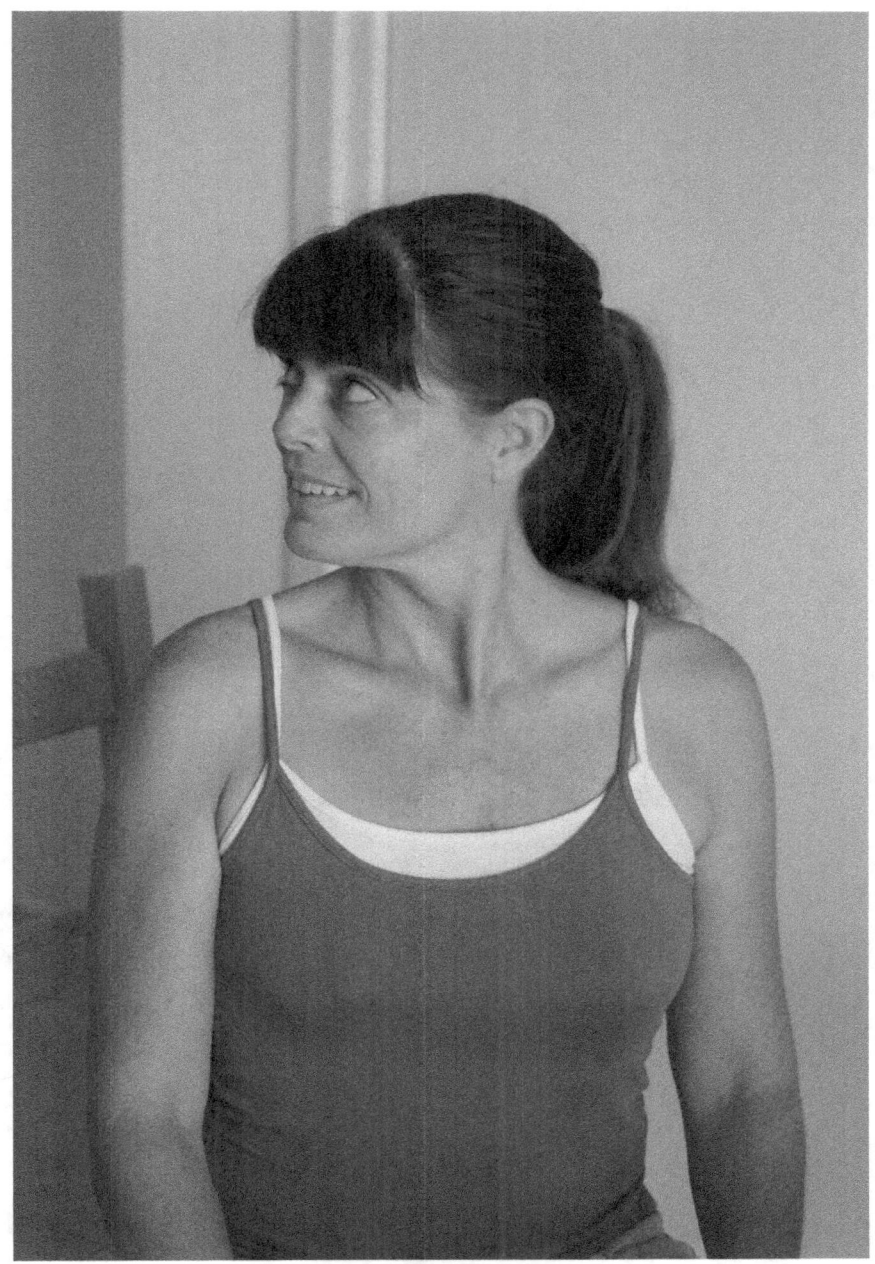

Exhale. Turn face left. ←

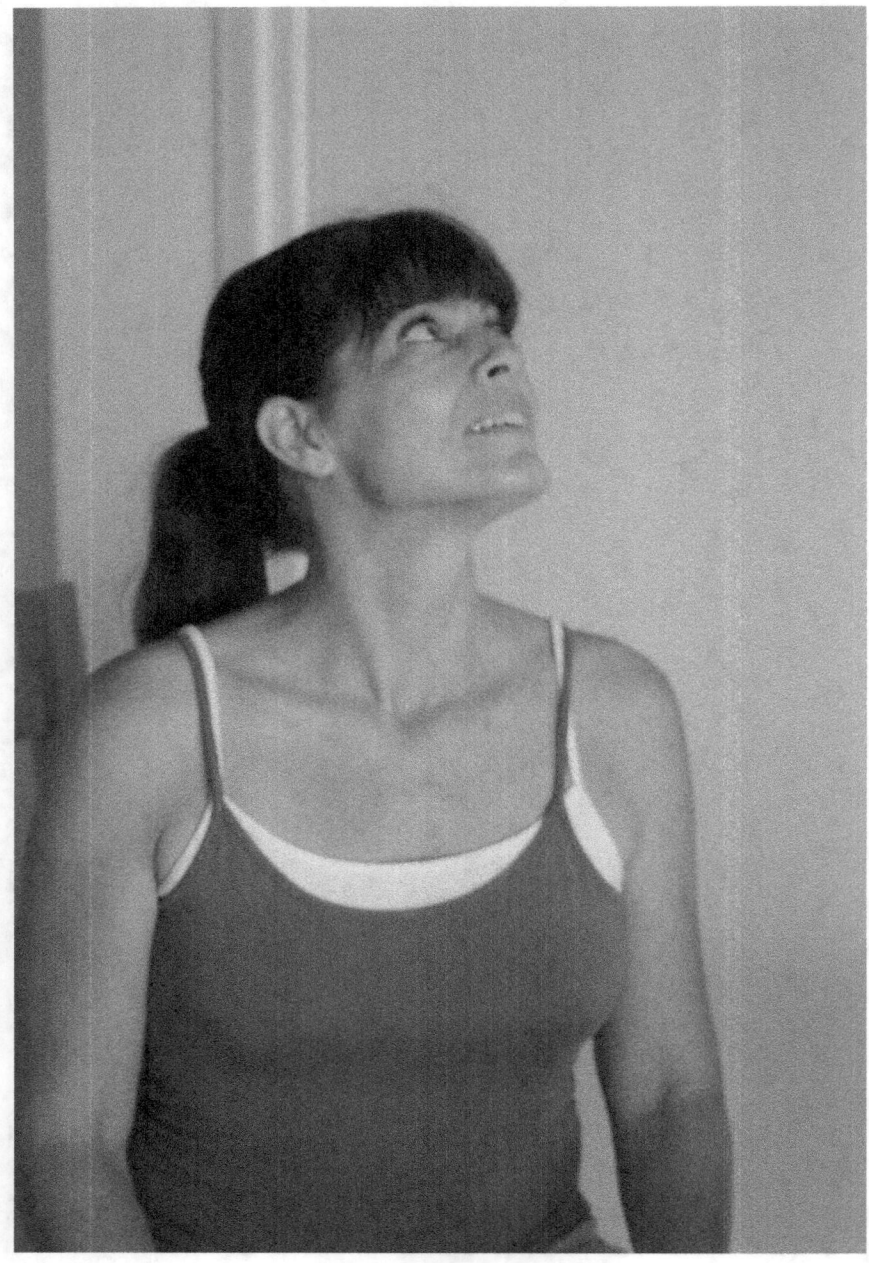

Inhale. Lift face up right. ↗

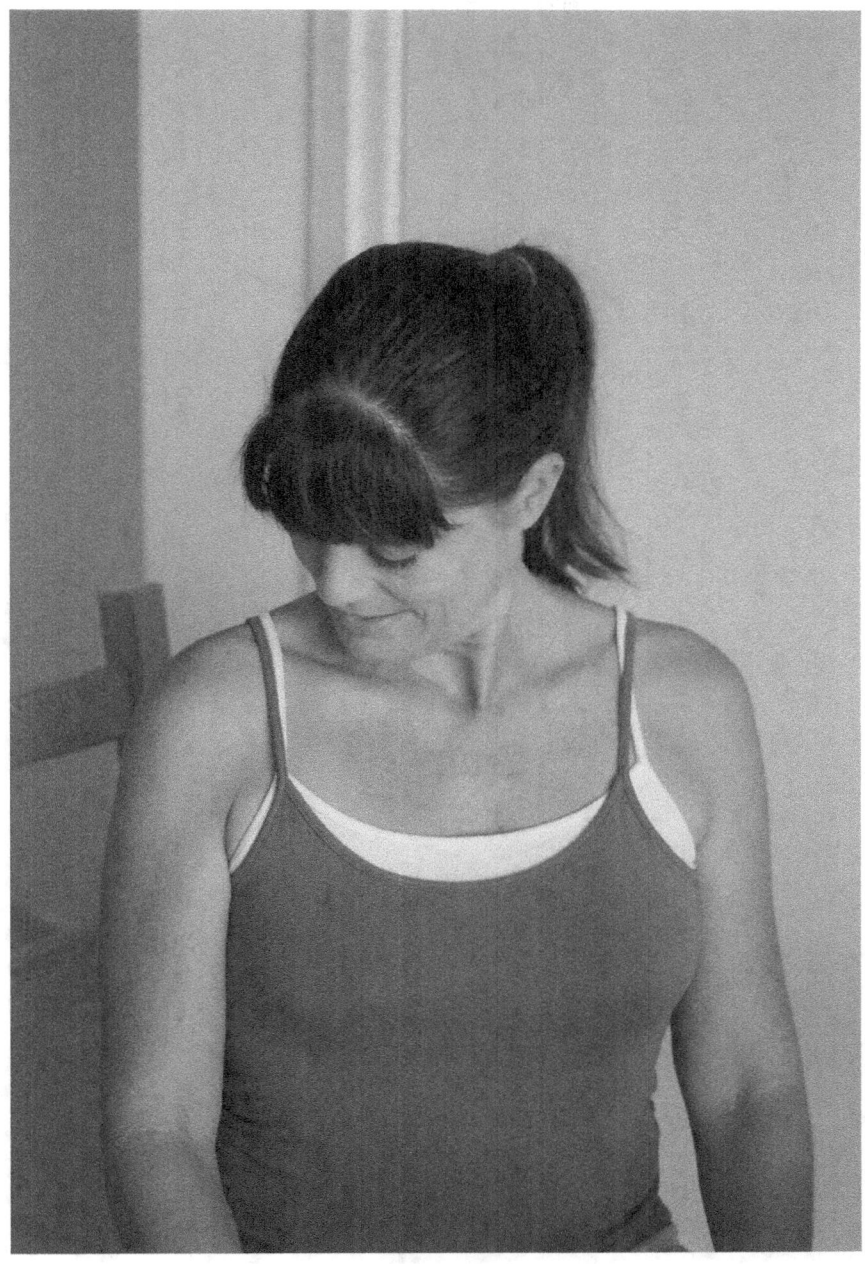

Exhale. Drop face down left. ↙

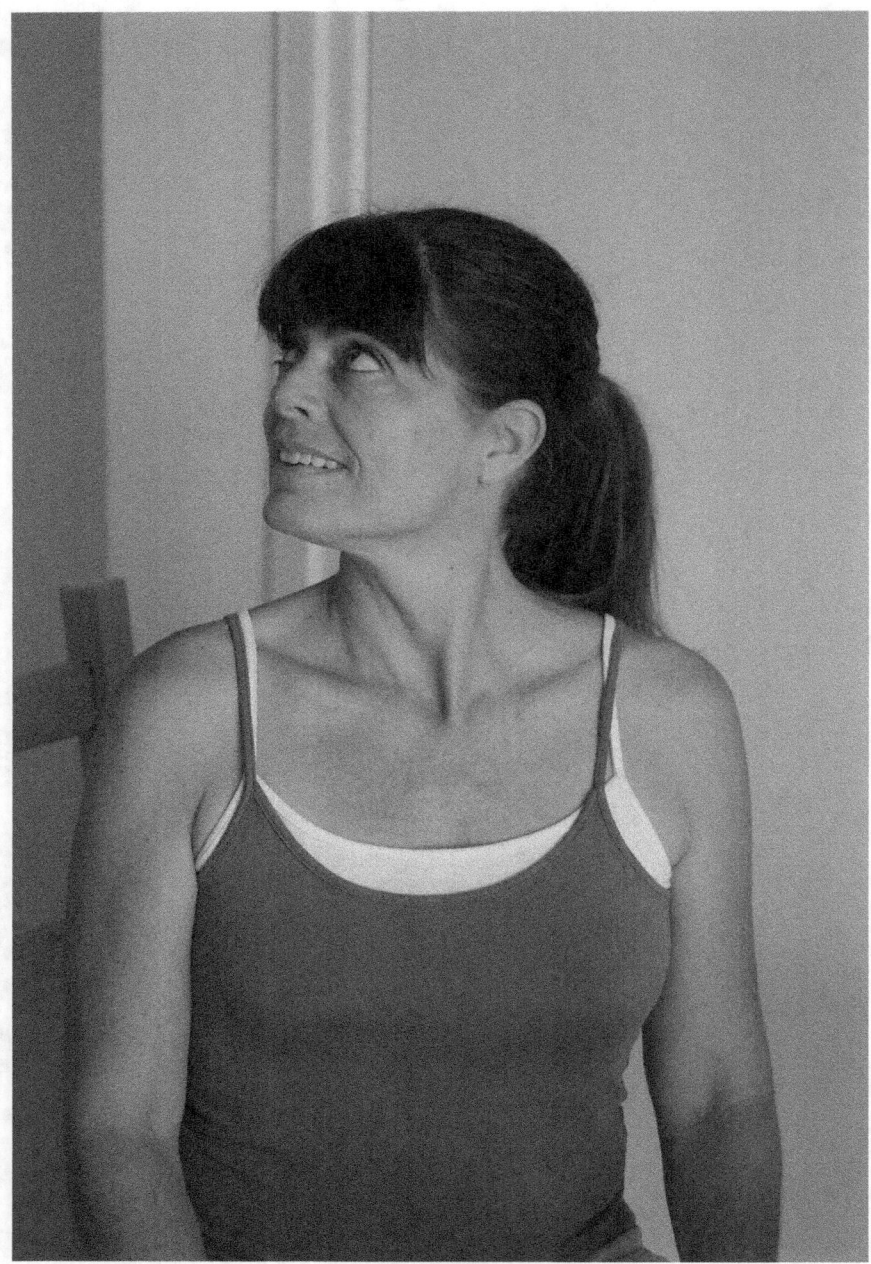

Inhale. Lift face up left. ↖

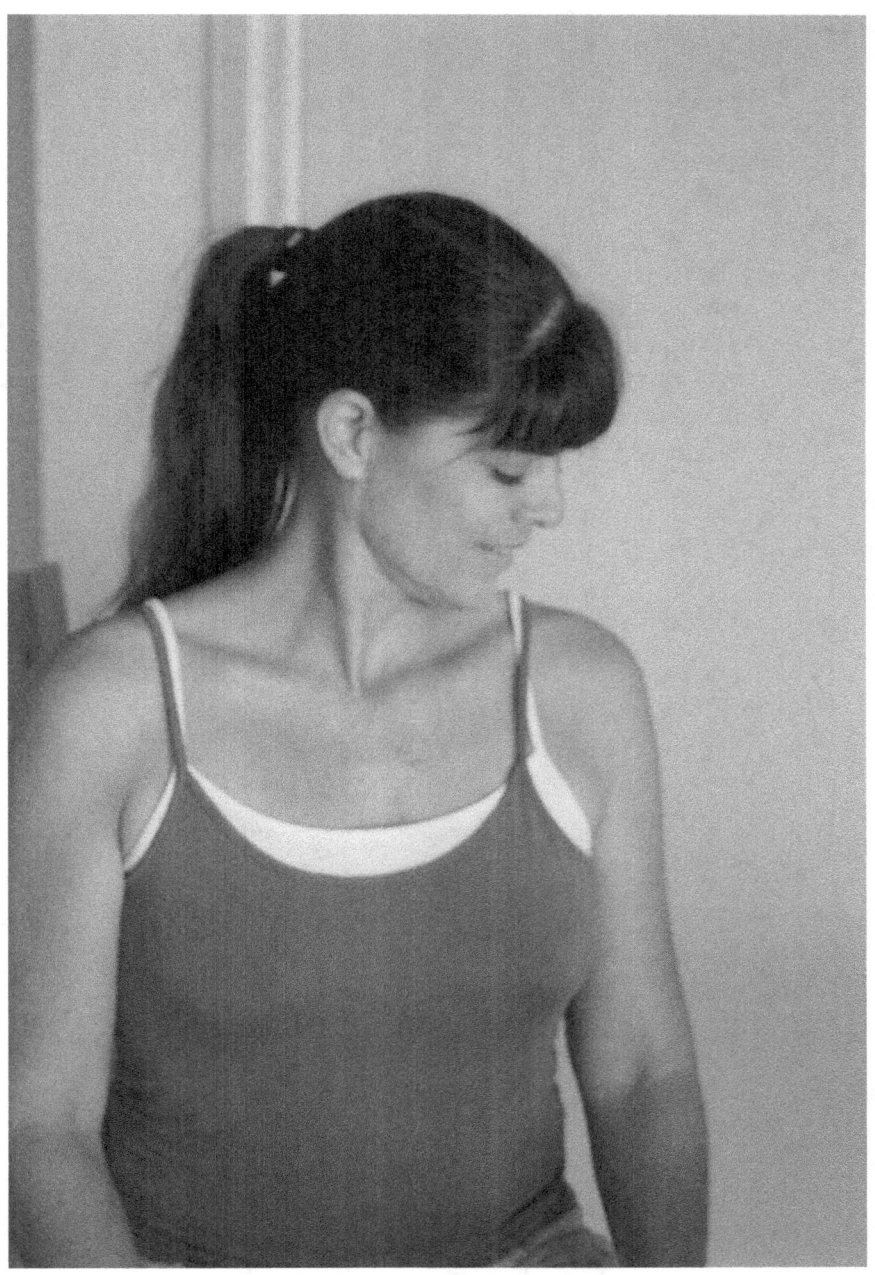

Exhale. Drop face down right. ↘

Benefits: *This relieves tension in the neck and shoulders, brings more blood flow to the brain and energizes the throat helping you to stay healthy and not as prone to sore throats. It also helps you to say what you need to say in difficult situations.*

3) **Side Stretch**
   - Place your right hand on the side of your seat or on the arm of your chair, depending on what kind of chair you have and what is more comfortable for you.
   - Inhale your left arm up beside your ear, keep it straight as you exhale and lean your whole upper body to the right. Imagine that you are smiling with the entire upper body. Add a smile on your face to make this posture easier.
   - Repeat on the other side.

Side Stretch

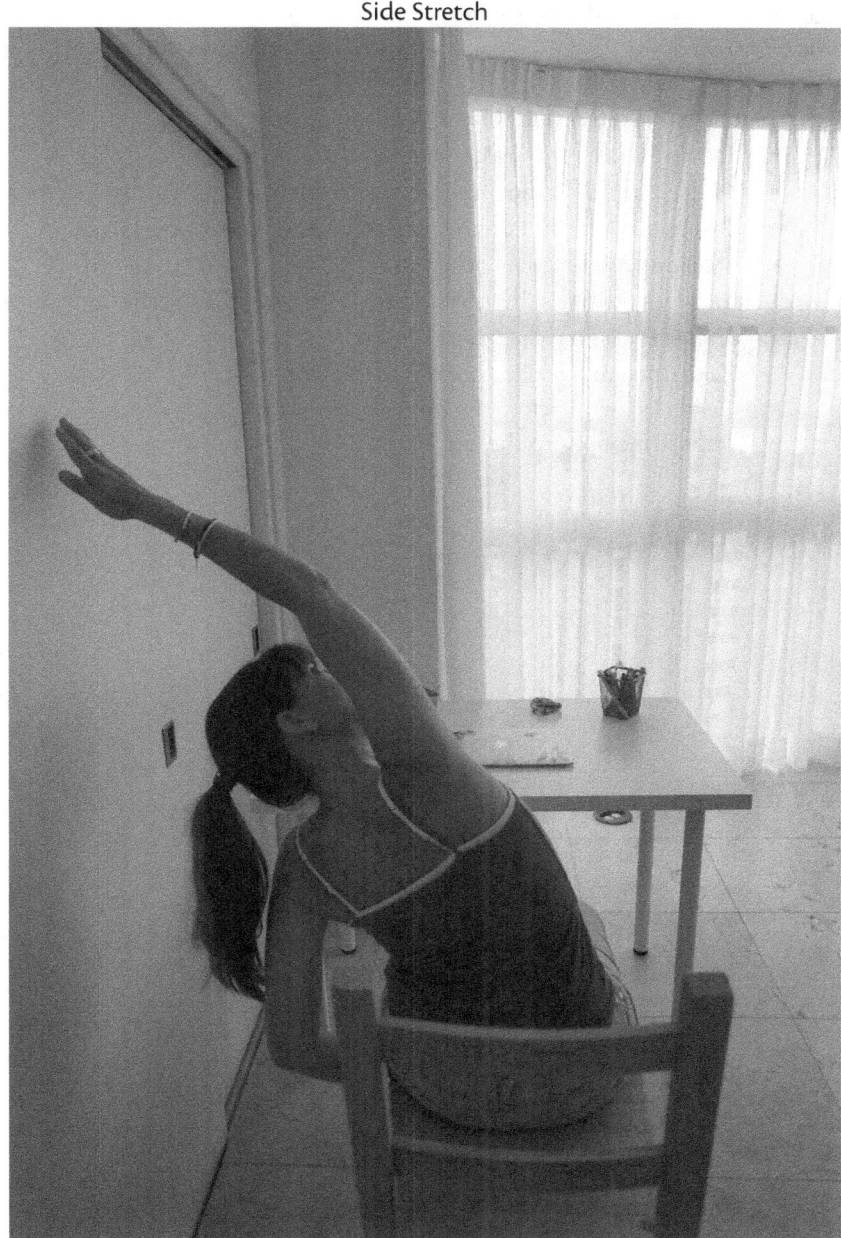

Lean to side. Support with one hand. Reach overhead with other hand.

Benefits: _This brings life and energy into your spine, nervous system and brain, stretches the side body and opens up the lungs, allowing you to breathe more deeply._

4) **Seated Half-Spinal Twist**
   - Inhale and sit very straight and tall.
   - Place your right hand on the arm of your chair or on the back of the seat.
   - Place your left hand on the outside of your right knee.
   - Inhale as you lengthen your spine.
   - Exhale, slowly twisting to your right, looking as far back over your right shoulder as is comfortably possible.
   - Take three to five deep breaths in the twist.
   - Release slowly back to the front on an exhale.
   - Repeat the twist to the left.

Seated Half-Spinal Twist

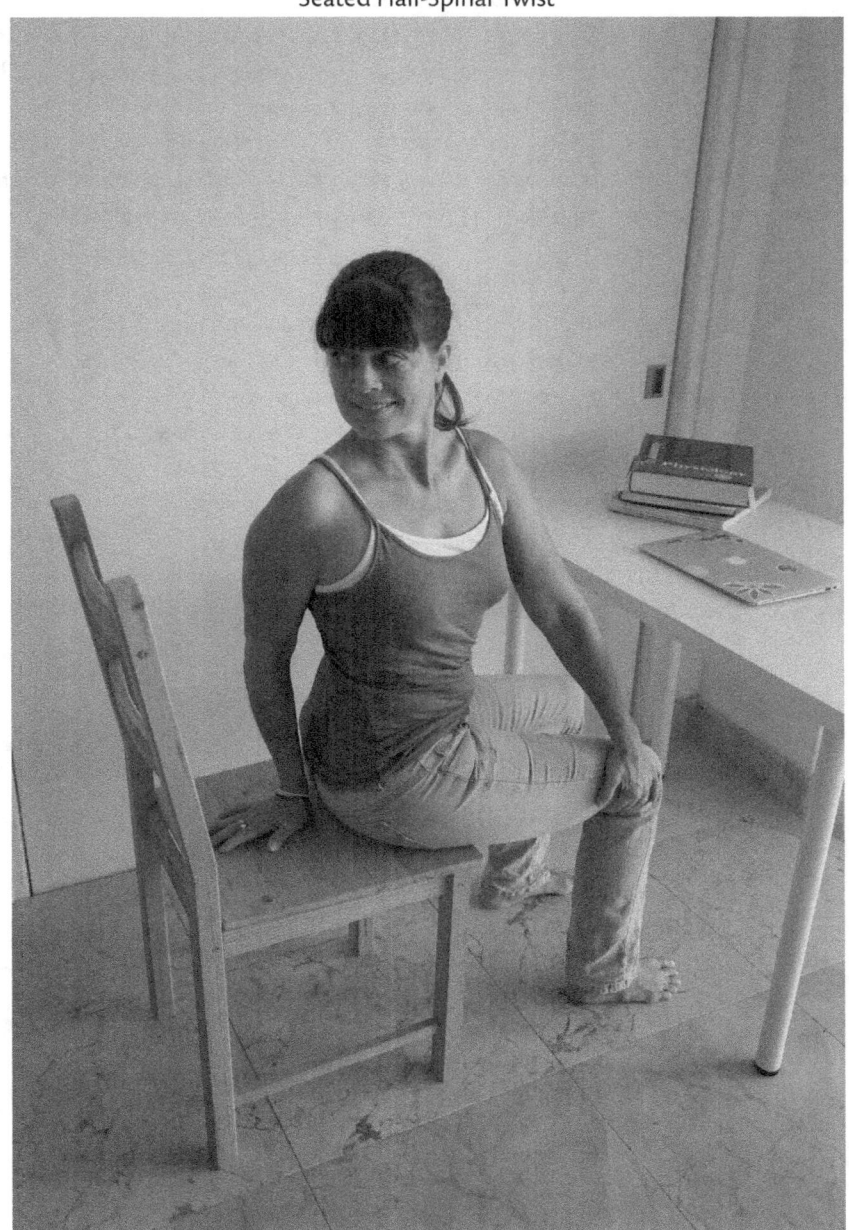

Sit on edge of chair. One hand behind. Turn to look over shoulder.

Benefits: This helps to bring energy and rejuvenation into your spine, so your entire nervous system is affected. It also helps your digestive system, which often gets sluggish from sitting and studying. It's important to keep the digestive organs toned and healthy. A healthy digestive system includes a healthy small intestine. According to Chinese Medicine, the small intestine helps us discern what are good choices in life. Keeping it healthy will help you make good study choices as well as good life choices. Also, a sluggish digestive system often creates sluggish thinking, which isn't very helpful when you are studying!

5) **Hip Opener**
- Seated in your chair, place your right ankle on your left knee. Let your right knee fall down towards the floor any amount that it will.
- Inhaling deeply reach your arms high up overhead.
- Straighten your elbows and spread your fingers wide apart.
- Exhale, fall forward over your right shin.
- Let your arms and head relax and hang towards the floor. If you are unable to bend this far forward, rest your arms or hands on your leg to support yourself, stretching further only when your body is ready.
- Hold for three to five breaths.
- Come up slowly on an inhale, and repeat on the other side.

Hip Opener

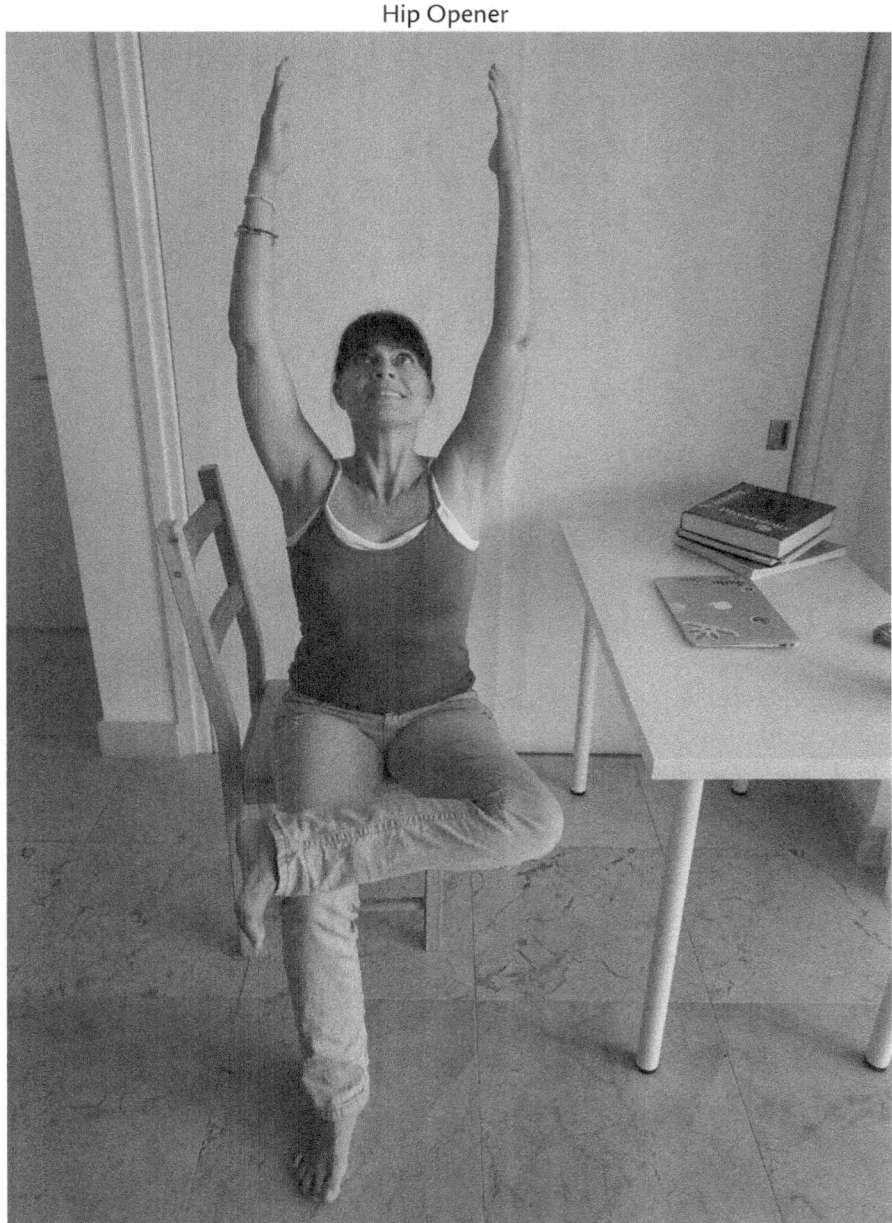

Sit on edge of chair. Opposite ankle on knee.

Hip Opener

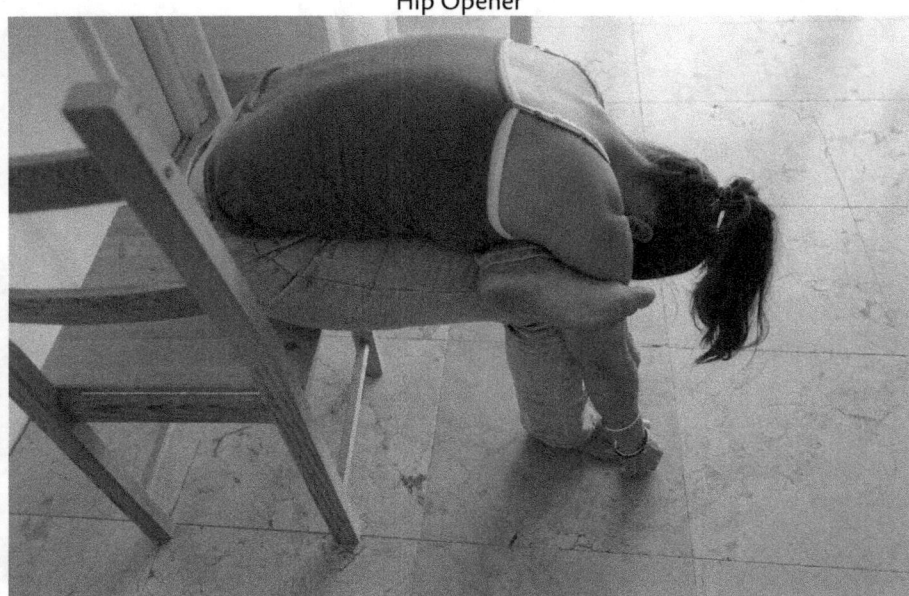

Bend forward.

Benefits: This releases tight, tense hips brought about by sitting, and releases pain and tension in the entire back, primarily the lower back. It also brings blood flow to the brain. You already know what the results of this are!

6) **Leg Refresher**
   - Slide back until your back is resting on the back of your chair.
   - Inhale, lift your feet from the floor and straighten your knees, keeping your toes pulled back toward your head.
   - Exhale, bend the knees, lower the feet to the floor.
   - Repeat ten to fifteen times.
   - For added challenge, remain seated on the edge of your chair as you lift your legs.
   - Be mindful to hold your abdominals in and keep your back straight.

Leg Refresher

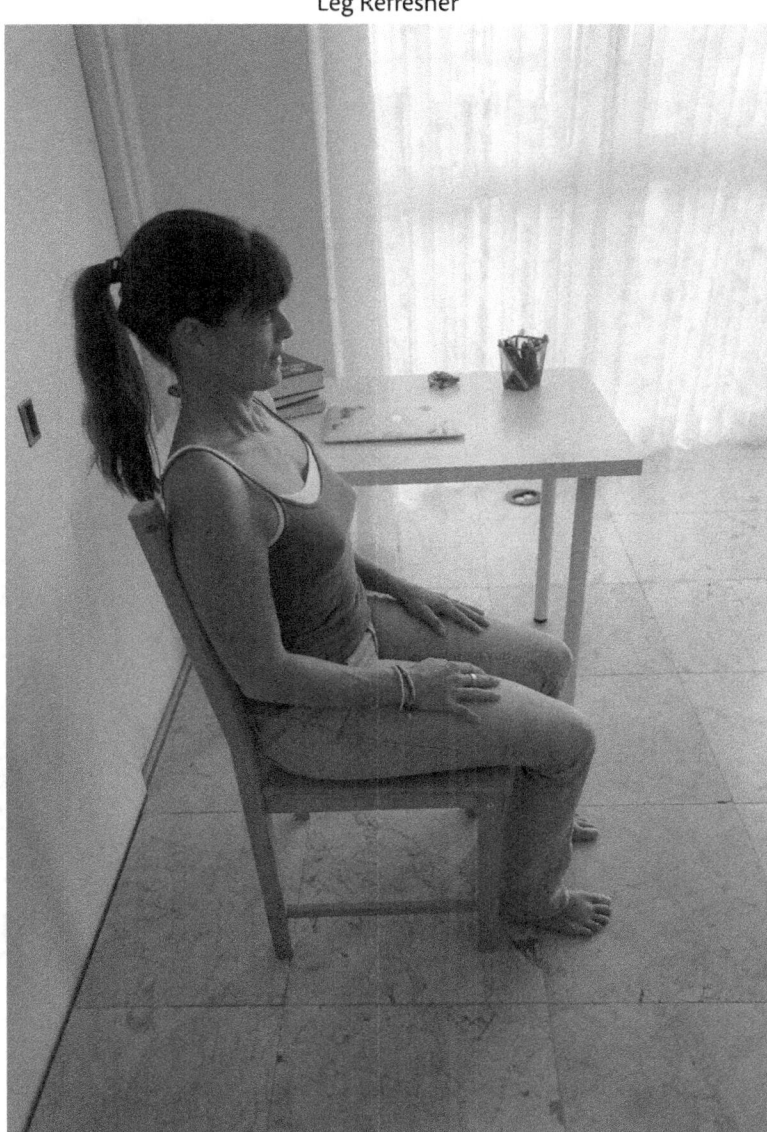

Inhale. Lift feet off floor.

Leg Refresher

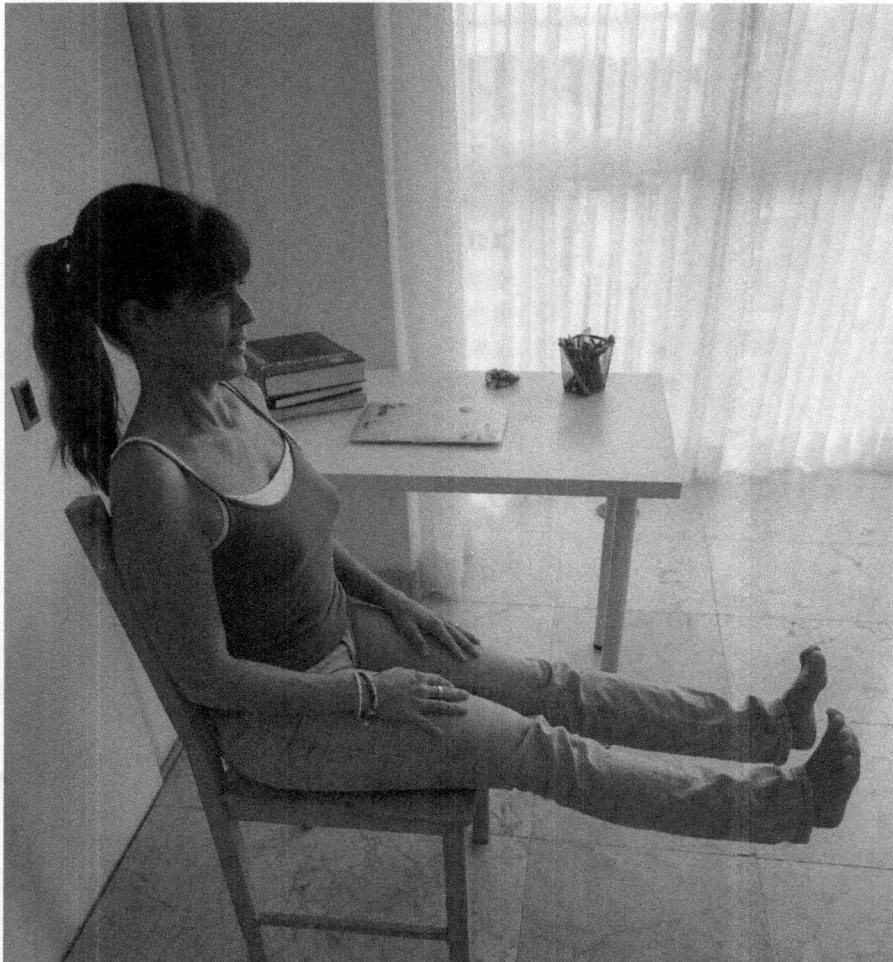

Exhale. Release feet down.

Benefits: *This keeps your leg muscles from atrophy and increases circulation to the lower extremities.*

7) **Restoring your Eyes, Part 1**
   - Inhale without moving your head at all, only move your eyes. Eyeballs look up toward the ceiling as far as you can.

- Exhale the eyes look down toward the floor as far as you can.
- Inhale the eyes up.
- Exhale the eyes down.
- Repeat 3-5 times.
- Inhale, look to the right as far as you can.
- Exhale, look to the left as far as you can.
- Repeat 3-5 times in each direction.
- Inhale look up to the right.
- Exhale, look down to the left. Eyes are moving diagonally.
- Repeat 3-5 times and then repeat the diagonal in the opposite direction.
- Now, breathing deeply, circle your eyes in giant circles around to the right 3-5 times, reverse and circle your eyes the opposite direction 3-5 times.

Restoring Your Eyes Part 2

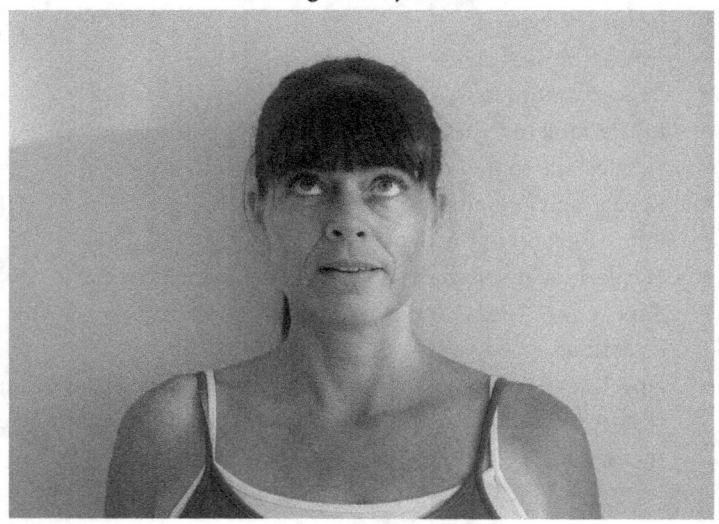

Inhale. Lift eyes up. ↑

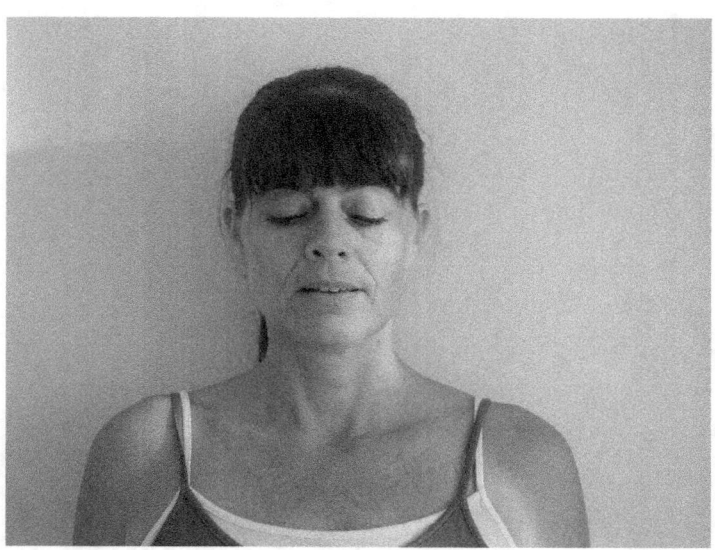

Exhale. Drop eyes down. ↓

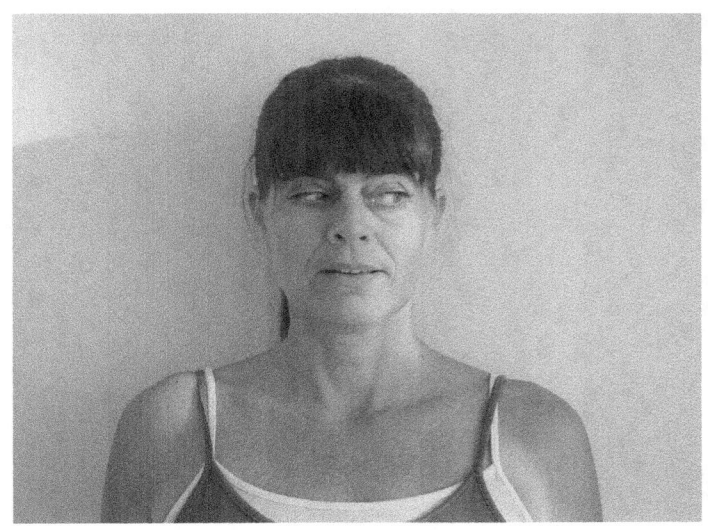

Inhale. Turn eyes right.➜

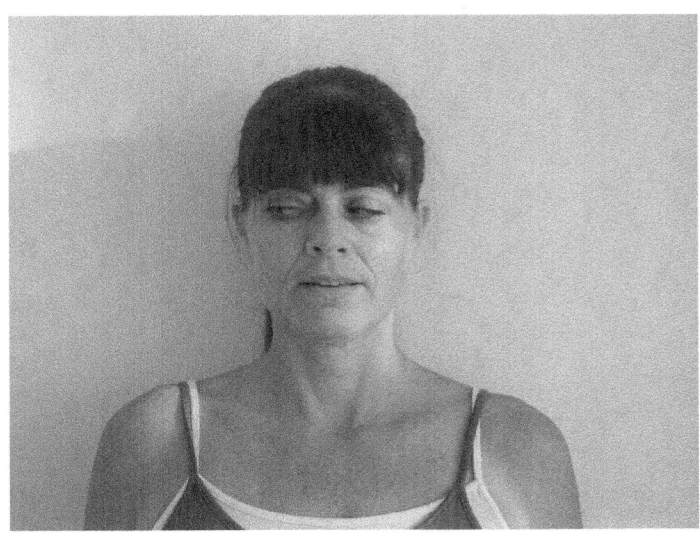

Exhale. Turn eyes left.←

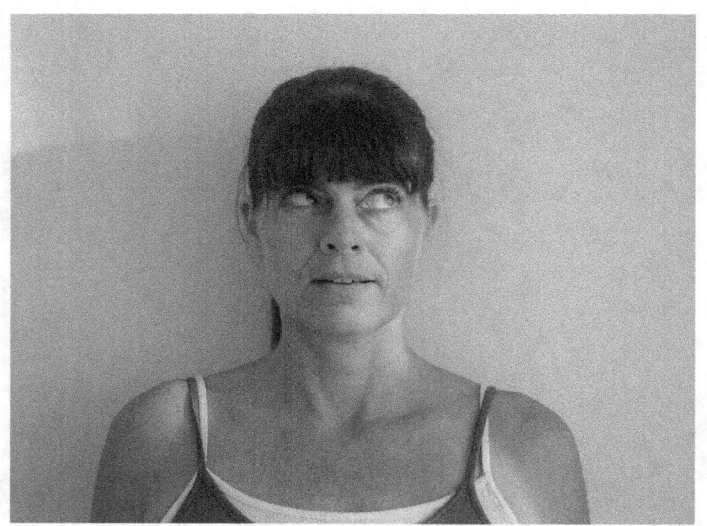

Inhale. Lift eyes up right. ⬈

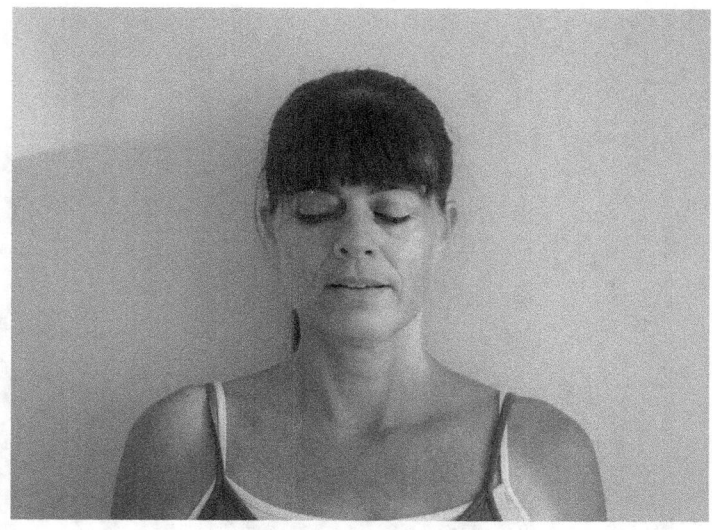

Exhale. Drop eyes down left. ⬋

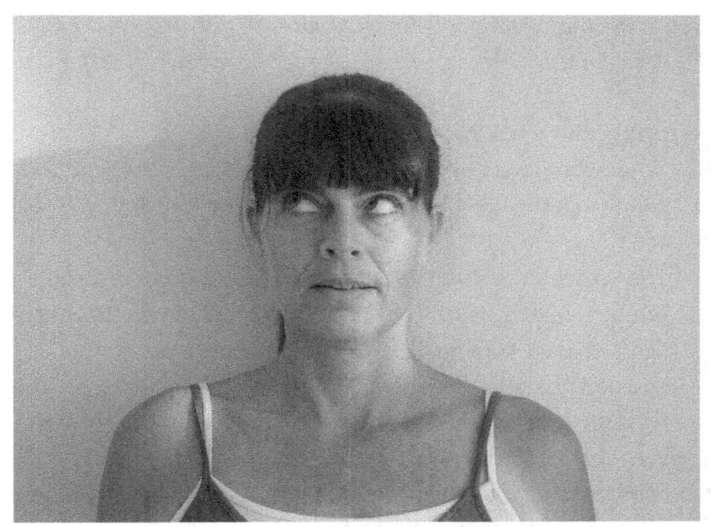

Inhale. Lift eyes up left. ↖

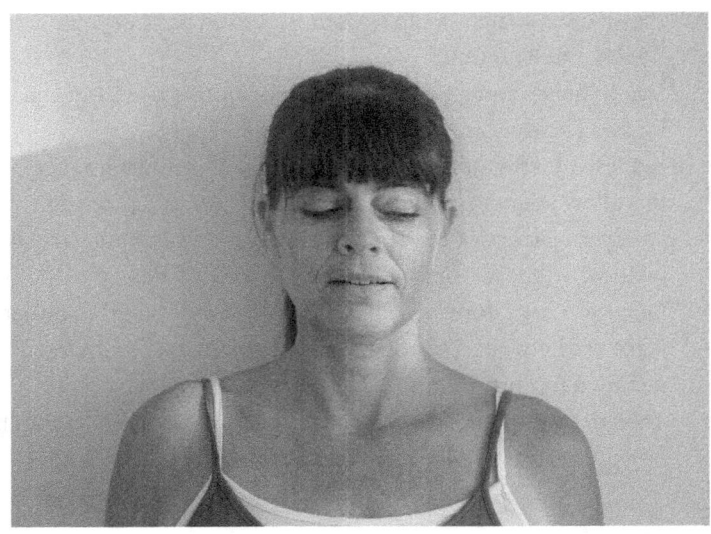

Exhale. Drop eyes down right. ↘

Benefits: The muscles of the eyes need exercise just like any other muscles. These exercises encourage you to use the full range of motion of your eye muscles and decreases eye strain and brain fog. Daily practice of eye exercises will keep your vision good for years to come.

8) **Restoring your Eyes, Part 2**
   - When you have finished the above exercises, close your eyes, rub your palms together very briskly, creating as much heat in your hands as you can.
   - Then place the palms of your hands right over your closed eyes.
   - Cut out all of the light. The eyes only rest fully when they are receiving no light, so make sure no light is getting to your eyes.
   - You don't have to press hard, just gently rest the fleshy part of your palm right on your eyelids. The warmth of the hands also seeps in around the eye muscles further relaxing the eyes.
   - Next, extend your right arm straight out in front of you at full length. Stick up your right thumb and look only at your right thumbnail.
   - Take a deep breath in and as you exhale, bring your right thumbnail in to touch the tip of your nose, while you continue to look at your nail.
   - Now as you inhale slowly extend your arm, all the way back out again until the elbow is straight, keeping your gaze fixed on your thumbnail only.
   - Repeat this 8-10 times.
   - Switch hands and look at your thumbnail, then look out the window, as far away as you can.
   - It doesn't matter whether you see what you're looking at very well or not.
   - Just allow your eyes to look as far away from you as possible.
   - Take your gaze back to your thumbnail, then take your gaze back out the window, to the farthest point you can look to. Repeat 8-10 times.
   - Once you have done this, once again, rub your palms together briskly.
   - Place the fleshy part of your palms over your eyes and allow your eyes to rest for a few breaths.
   - Then drop your chin to your chest, release your hands to your lap, slowly open your eyes and let them come to focus.

Restoring Your Eyes Part 2

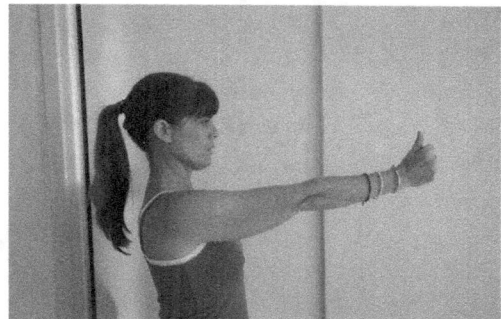

Extend arm, look at thumb.

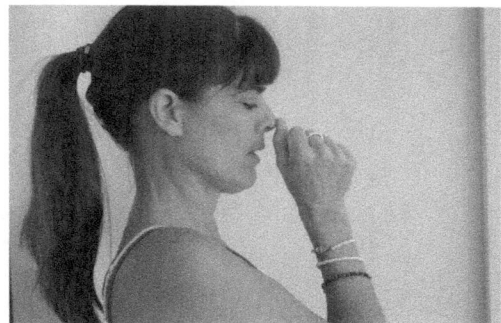

Bring thumb to nose. Watch thumb.

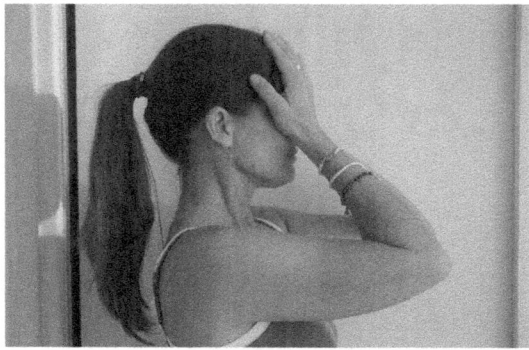

Rub hands together. Place palms over eyes

Benefits: These eye exercises will help keep your eyes healthy. Muscles of the eyes need exercise just like any other muscles. These exercises encourage you to use the full range of motion of your eye muscles, which decreases eye strain and brain fog. Daily practice of eye exercises will keep your vision good for years to come. They help prevent eye fatigue as well as degenerative eye conditions such as nearsightedness. When the eyes are feeling strong and clear, it is difficult to have brain fog. Exercising your eyes will help you to think clearly as well as see clearly.

Asana Notes

Asana Notes

Asana Notes

Asana Notes

CHAPTER 5
The Breath

"Breath is the key to ultimate emancipation."
—HATHA YOGA PRADIPIKA

The Hatha Yoga Pradipika tells us that the mind is the king of the senses, and the breath is the king of the mind. So now that you have released your body with asana, let's think about the second step of our three-step system: the breath.

In yoga, the breathing exercises are usually referred to as "pranayama." "Prana" means life force. It is not referring to the oxygen we breathe, but rather, the life we get from that oxygen. "Yama" means control, so "pranayama" is loosely translated as "breath control." It is said in yoga that when we learn to control the breath, we then gain control, or mastery, over the mind.

Since the main goal of pranayama is to give you mastery over the mind, let's look at some simple breathing techniques to help you listen, study, and learn.

How to Start Your Breathing Practice

1) Find a comfortable quiet place where you can practice your breathing.

As you become more and more proficient, you can do your breath work any place you like. I recommend lying down to breathe as you're learning. But if that's not possible, the second best option is seated on the floor with your back supported by the wall. A chair is another option, but as a last resort since we're focusing on getting your body out of a chair shape as often as possible.

2) Observe your breathing.

Begin by making yourself as comfortable as possible so that you can get acquainted with your own breathing patterns. Observe if breathing is very easy or challenging for you. Close your eyes and notice. Do you breathe naturally through your nose or your mouth? Do you feel your breath constricted anywhere? Do you breathe down into your belly? Do you breathe into your chest? Do you hold your breath after you inhale or after you exhale? What else do you notice about your breath?

3) Move on to the pranayama of your choice.

Once you take a few moments to observe and acquaint yourself with your natural breathing patterns, move on to the pranayama of your choice. Keep in mind your natural breathing patterns may be different each time you check in. This is because our breathing is affected by what's happening inside of us and around us. Regular practice of these pranayama exercises may very likely change your day to day breathing patterns.

We will begin with the most basic breathing technique and build from there. Once you are accustomed to doing the breathing, or pranayama, then you can choose to do any one you wish.

Just as in the previous chapter, there are blank pages at the end of this chapter. Use them to keep notes for yourself. Track your progress and clarify for yourself the shifts you feel from the breathing exercises. As you did with the asanas write down, on a scale of 1-10, how you feel before doing pranayama exercises and after doing them. 1 will represent feeling your worst and 10 will represent feeling your best. Taking time to note which breathing technique you did will help you, in the future, to remember which one worked most optimally for you. That may stay the same or it may change. In either case it is useful to know how we change or stay the same over time.

Pranayama:

CAUTION: If you feel dizzy or lightheaded at any time when practicing pranayama, stop the exercise immediately. Return to normal breathing and allow your body to return to its normal state.

Pranayama #1 Circular Breathing:
This is not the same circular breath as used by the people who play wind instruments. This is the yogic circular breath.

- Find your comfortable position, inhale and exhale evenly through the nose only. Breathe this way for a few rounds to get comfortable with it.
- Once you are accustomed to that, begin to count the length of your breath. If possible, begin to inhale for four counts and exhale four counts. If that is too long for you try beginning on a two-count and move up to a four count. Once you're comfortable with four counts, then you can move up to six counts, eight counts, ten counts, whatever is comfortable for you.
- Now that you're comfortable counting and making the inhale and the exhale the same length, try to remove any pauses at the end of the inhale and the end of the exhale. This is Circular Breathing.

Circular Breathing

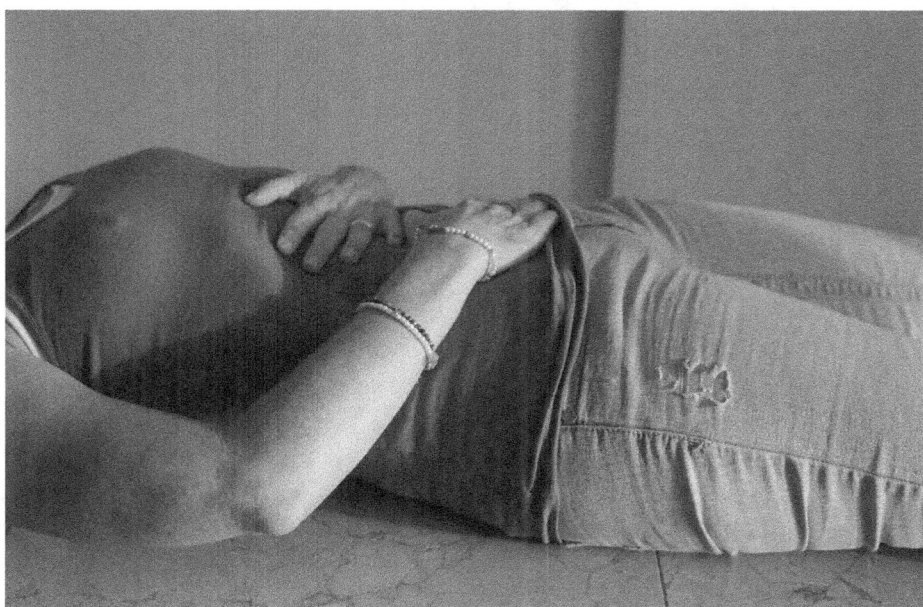

Inhale and exhale without pausing.

Benefits: This increases energy, eliminates stress, anxiety, and depression, and is deeply relaxing. It can awaken creative energies as well as build the immune system and alleviate pain. It may be beneficial in preventing injury and illness as well as recovering from injury and illness.

Pranayama #2 Three-part or Complete Breath, Deerga Swasam Pranayama

- Place one hand on your upper belly and one hand on your lower belly. Breathing deeply in through your nose, expand the lower belly first, then the upper belly or diaphragm area, then your chest, then exhale through the nose. Repeat as many times as you like.
- In the beginning it may be wise to do this only three to five times because you may not be accustomed to taking in such high volumes of breath.

Three-Part or Complete Breath

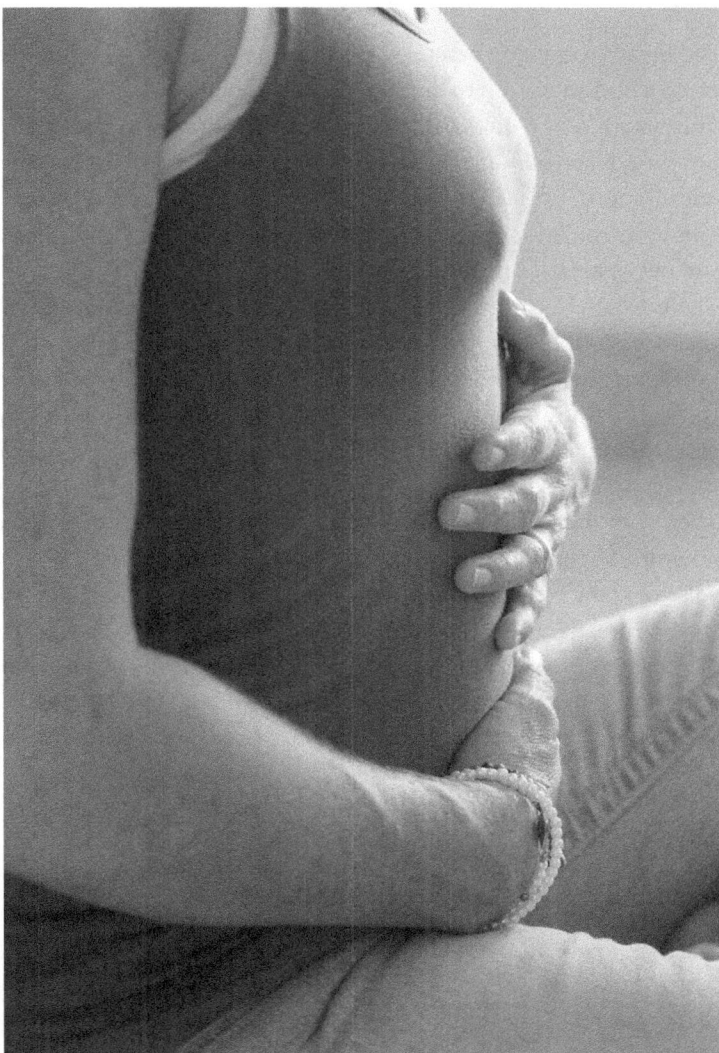

Inhale. Expand lower belly, upper belly, then chest.

Benefits: This teaches you to breathe fully which increases your oxygen level, bringing greater health to your entire body and decreases stress and anxiety, bringing your awareness to the present moment and calming your mind.

Pranayama #3 – Bee Breath or Bhramari Pranayama

- Bee breath should be practiced on an empty stomach. Once you learn how to do it, it is suggested to do three to nine rounds.
- This breath also requires inhaling and exhaling through the nose. However, on the exhale you hum the letter 'm' like "mmmm," giving this technique a vocalization.
- You want to continue the "mmm" sound for as long as you can. When you run out of breath, inhale and repeat.
- There are specific positions, or mudras, for the hands in Bee Breath. You can practice it without hand positions and it is still quite effective. Using the hand positions, however, will make it even more powerful. Both hands do the same thing. The thumb will go just inside the tragus, the flap at the front of your external ear where you have that little bit of cartilage, not too forcefully, just enough to close off the ears.
- Then your index and middle fingers will rest on top of your closed eyelids, your ring finger will rest just at the edge of your nostril, and your pinky finger will rest at the edge of your mouth. Once you have both hands in place, begin the bee breath by inhaling through the nose, exhaling through the nose and humming the "mmm" sound. You may continue until you feel yourself calm and relaxed. Then return to your normal breathing.

Bee breath

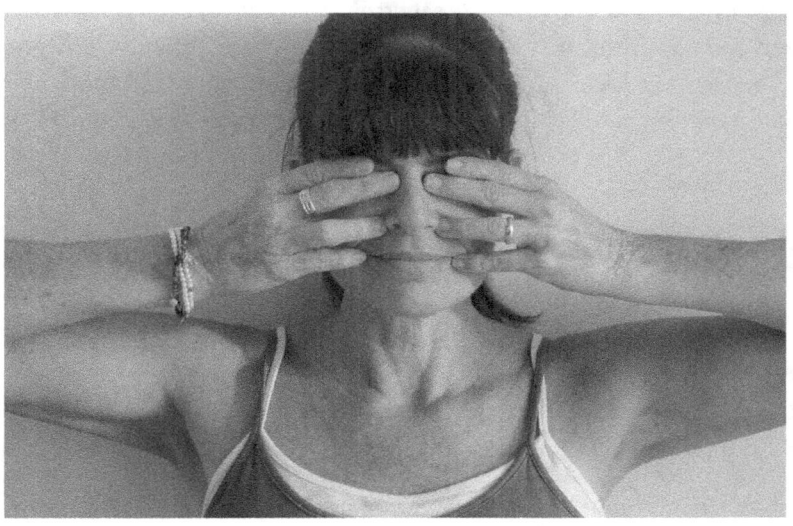

Hands in position.

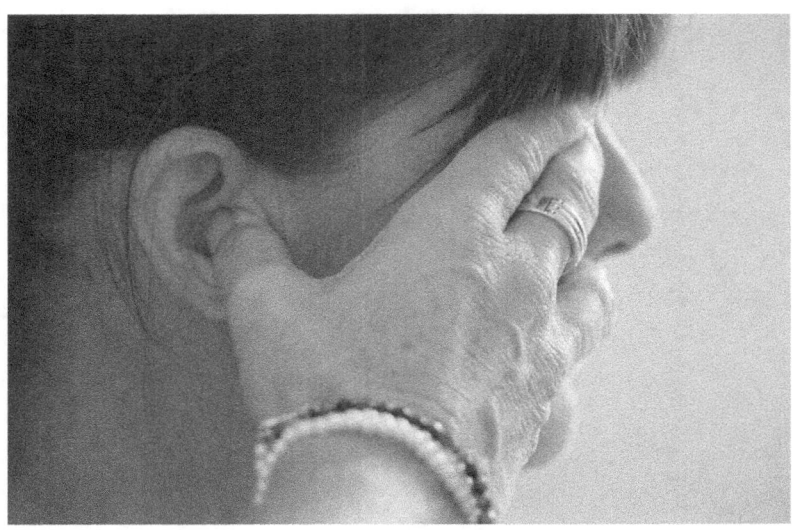

Inhale through nose. Exhale sound mmm...

Benefits: _Very good for calming your mind. It's one of the best to relieve your mind of agitation, frustration, or anxiety and to get rid of anger. It helps get rid of slight headaches and improves concentration and memory. Who doesn't need that when they're studying? It has also been said to stop anxiety attacks as it produces extreme calm and bliss. I have had a number of students verify that it has in fact stopped panic attacks for them._

Pranayama Notes

Pranayama Notes

Pranayama Notes

Pranayama Notes

CHAPTER 6
The Mind

"By drawing our senses of perception inward, we are able to experience the control, silence, and quietness of the mind."
~ B.K.S IYENGAR

Your Mind: Friend Or Foe?

Now you have learned the foundation of how to keep your body more comfortable by breaking up your study time with specific movements (or asanas) from Chapter 4, designed to keep your circulation moving, your spine supple and your joints flexible. You then layered on breathing techniques which oxygenate your blood and organs and also refresh your mind while simultaneously calming your nervous system. It is now time to shift your focus to the mind.

By now you may have noticed a lessening of what Buddhists call "monkey mind." This is when the mind jumps quickly from one idea to another and can't focus on anything for long. Breaking up sedentary activities, like studying, with movement makes your body more comfortable. This way the mind doesn't constantly jump to thoughts of discomfort in the body. As we learned from the Hatha Yoga Pradipikipa, the breath is the master of the mind. In other words, the mind can be controlled by controlling the breath. You probably became aware of the mind calming, slowing down and focusing more by doing the breathing exercises in Chapter 5.

Now it's time to use the mind to accomplish what you need to more effectively. Do you pay attention to your thoughts? I mean really pay attention to the script that runs through your head? We all have a constant dialogue or conversation playing, whether we are always aware of it or not. Do you ever think, or say aloud, things like: "There's no way I'm going to pass that test," or, "I'm never going to finish this project on time ?"

These kinds of thoughts may seem harmless and even seem like reality because we have all of the facts to prove that they are accurate. But it is exactly this kind of thinking that is like an enemy that sabotages you and can leave you exactly where you don't want to be: failing a test and with an unfinished project at the time of your deadline! Shift that type of thinking immediately. It does not serve your higher purpose of graduating with ease and it is like cancer. It just keeps growing if left unchecked. The more of these types of thoughts you have, the more of them you will continue to have. You will end up feeling like a salmon swimming upstream throughout your entire college career and beyond into your work career.

The exercise that follows can apply to anything you need to do. Pass an exam with flying colors, complete a project, graduate or ace a job interview. There's no end to what you can use this technique to accomplish. Get creative and try it for anything you like. The more you use it, the better you will get at becoming the architect of your life as you create a blueprint for everything you need or want to accomplish. We will do a visualization to set you on a clear path of how to achieve a desired result.

Visualization is a type of meditation, but in my personal experience, the two differ somewhat. Visualization has a definite beginning and end, whereas meditation has neither. It doesn't begin or end. It's like you have stepped into a vast cosmos of timelessness and stepped back out again when you are done. But the meditation hasn't actually stopped nor did it begin when you arrived. It was, is, and always will be there.

First, get very clear about what you want to visualize into actual existence. The more clear and specific you are the more effective you will be. For our purposes, I will use the example of passing your final exam in calculus with a 98 percent or above. But for your own purpose, you can substitute the calculus exam for whatever you need it to be.

Use the blank pages at the end of this chapter to write down, in very specific detail, what you want to visualize. The more details you write, and the more specific they are, the better. This exercise is very important to write down because writing it will strengthen your ability to bring it to fruition. You are the architect of your life and this is your blueprint.

Creating Your Reality Visualization

- Get into a comfortable position, but not one in which you are likely to fall asleep.
- Close your eyes and take a few deep full breaths.
- See, feel or imagine yourself taking your calculus test and notice that it is effortless. You know how to solve every problem easily.
- Now see, feel, or imagine yourself handing in your test.
- Notice how you feel after you have completed your test successfully. How does your body feel? How does your mind feel?
- Notice now what you are thinking about yourself. What do you say to others about yourself and your test? Hear what you say. Then hear what others have to say about you and your performance on your test.
- Look at your posture. Notice how you look, as you hear what you say, and when you hear what others say about you. Notice how others look at you.
- Now see, feel or imagine yourself learning your grade on your test. See, feel or imagine that you got a 98, 99, or a 100 on your exam.
- How does it make you feel in your body?
- What are you thinking? What do you say about your grade to others? How do you see your body? How do you see yourself? How do others look at you when you tell them your grade? What do others say to you about your grade? What do other people say to each other about your grade?
- Now notice, what is the taste of making this really high grade on your exam? Just the same as we sometimes experience something wonderful and say something like, "that was a sweet experience!". What is the taste of this really high grade you just received on your test? Experience that taste.
- And now what is the smell of that grade? Just the same as when you land a new job and you know you're going to make more money, you say, "oh, it's the smell of money, I smell the money." What is the smell of this really high grade on your test?
- Take time to go through all of your senses in relationship to the results of the grade that you want to receive on your test. See the grade, see it written on the paper, or on the computer screen or wherever you receive it.

See how you look. Notice how it feels to receive the grade. Hear what you say and what you think. And what others say and think about you. Taste that taste of success, of victory. Smell the smell of that success, of that victory. Allow yourself to take a few slow deep breaths, and absorb everything you see, hear, feel, taste, and smell about this wonderful grade that you made. Allow it to sink in, and then offer up your gratitude for that wonderful grade. Say thank you. It doesn't have to be to anyone or anything. Just gratitude. Allow yourself to feel the gratitude. Allow yourself to offer the gratitude. Now open your eyes and know that now you have seen, heard, felt, tasted and smelled the experience. It is in place and ready to become your reality.

Reality Visualization Blueprint

Reality Visualization Blueprint

Reality Visualization Blueprint

Reality Visualization Blueprint

CHAPTER 7
Successful Graduation and Beyond

"To me, the sign of success is a smile. The number of smiles that one has in their day-to-day life indicates how successful one is. You may have a big bank balance, a lot of money. But if you can't smile, if you are tensed, upset, angry, would you call such a person successful?"
~ SRI SRI RAVI SHANKAR

How do you measure success? Look back at our original thoughts at the beginning of this book about what a successful yoga practice is. Many of you probably thought a successful yoga practice meant being able to perform all of the asanas or postures in a hatha yoga practice with ease. You may have never thought about the possibility that a successful yoga practice would be using the simplest aspects of yoga to attain your goals of good grades and graduating from school! But as you have seen and experienced through the use of this book, a successful yoga practice can be exactly that.

Just as you probably redefined your idea of what yoga is you may also be able to redefine your idea of what success is. Practicing yoga throughout your college career will help you to look at everything in the world around you with a more open mind.

I encourage you to use the simple tools you learned in this book to help you with all of your school and life challenges. Once you make them a habit you won't have to even think about it. You will automatically know what to do.

Take a moment to review the three powerful tools we learned in the pages of this book. Body, Mind and Breath. What a powerful combination! It is unbeatable, and using the Body, Mind, Breath Connection, you will be unbeatable too. You now possess the tools you need to give you an edge and keep your skills sharp. Please use them and share them with everyone you know. I believe it is everyone's right to know how to use their body, their mind and their breath to the fullest capacity. It is unnecessary to go through life not knowing how to optimize the possibilities you have as a part of you.

Your body is your precious vehicle that takes you from place to place. It is imperative that you take care of that vehicle so that you remain happy in it for as long as you have it. After all, you can't take it back to the dealer and get a new one. Use your breath to keep your vehicle running smoothly and use your mind to create the roadmap for where you want to go. If we all can master the use of these tools we can do anything. Imagine a world full of people who all know the secrets you have learned in this book and all use them daily.

Now that you have learned how to do the physical postures, the breath and the visualization, let's take a moment to review what you need to do to use yoga while you study.

The Body, Mind, Breath Connection Formula to Graduate with Ease and Maintain Health:

- Set your alarm to sound just before your brain loses focus
- Stop what you're doing and do any of the physical movements you learned in this book, or any others you know
- Notice when you feel stressed or anxious
- Do one or more of the breathing exercises in this book to restore your calm
- Visualize the outcome you want in any situation using as many of your 5 senses as you can.

It really is as easy as the steps you've learned in this book. Now go grab the tiger by the tail, conquer the world and fly as high as you want. I know you can do it!

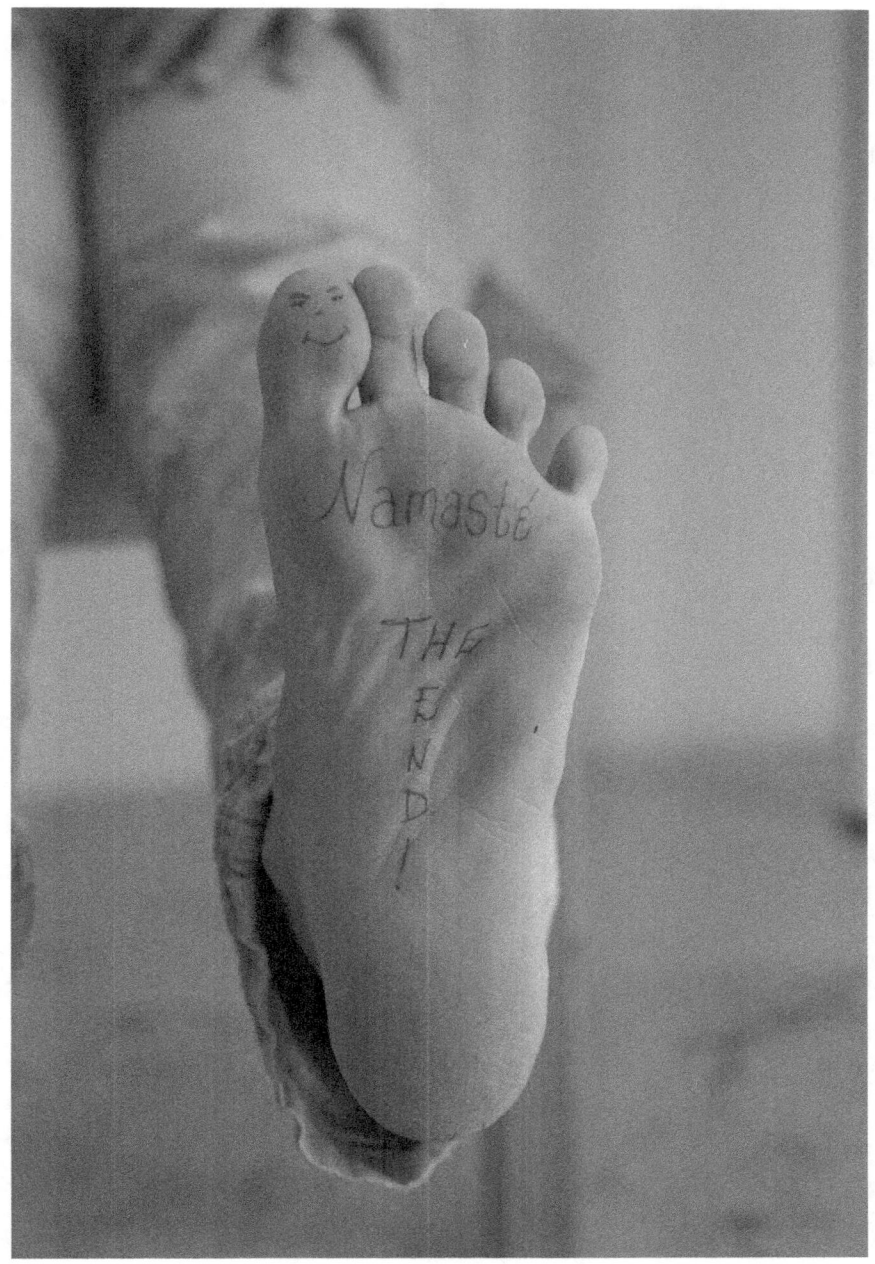

Index

www.ingramcontent.com/pod-product-compliance
Lightning Source LLC
Chambersburg PA
CBHW070203290526
45789CB00002B/887